TO YOUR HEALTH

*A Lifestyle of Health,
Happiness and Confidence*

By
ESTHER AVANT

To Your Health: A Lifestyle of Health, Happiness, and Confidence

Printed in the United States of America

Hardcover ISBN: 978-1-960876-67-6
Paperback ISBN: 978-1-960876-68-3
Ebook ISBN: 978-1-960876-69-0

Library of Congress Control Number: 2024912078

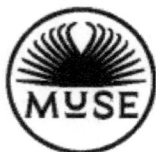

Muse Literary

To help you implement everything
you'll learn in this book, I've created a portal
of additional resources, including worksheets
for all the journaling prompts and written exercises,
a sample workout program, and more.

Scan the code below with your smartphone
or go to www.estheravant.com/book-portal-signup
to access it all!

AUTHOR'S NOTE

The clients in this book are largely amalgams of several clients. Names and recognizable details have been changed to protect their anonymity. Conversations have been recalled from notes and memory.

This book is not intended as a substitute for the medical or mental health advice of physicians or mental health professionals. The reader should consult a physician or therapist in matters relating to his/her physical or mental health and particularly with respect to any symptoms that may require diagnosis or medical attention.

DEDICATION

To Mom.

The career I've chosen and the woman
I've become is due—in no small part—to you.
I wish you were here, but I know you'd be proud.

TABLE OF CONTENTS

NOTE TO READER

This is not a diet book.

If you're looking for another book filled with lists of what not to eat, a dozen variations of green smoothies, and 60 pages of exercise descriptions, this ain't it.

I wrote this book for my mom.

I wrote this book for you.

I wrote this book for your mom.

I wrote this book for any woman who's ever said she wants to be healthier, feel better about herself, have more energy, be more confident, or yeah, have her clothes fit better.

Of course, this book *can* help you lose weight—if that's your goal—but it will also help you do so much more than that.

If you *do* want to lose weight, this book will help you do it more successfully: with less restriction, deprivation, overwhelm, and shame—and results you're confident can last a lifetime.

But you don't *have* to want to lose weight in order for this book to be for you. (And while I do refer to weight loss throughout the book, just know that the broader principles apply to any health goal you have.)

You deserve to exist in the world in whatever body you want. You'll find that the Gone For Good formula I'm teaching you in this book is applicable to a wider range of health goals, as well as nearly *any* lifestyle goal you may want to pursue, and will help you live your healthiest, happiest, and most confident life.

You may already have some idea of what you "should" be doing in order to reach your goals. If not, we're going to cover the most important health and weight-loss habits in a way that's simple, straightforward, and helps you cut through all the confusion and misinformation about exercise and nutrition.

Having worked in the fitness and health industry for nearly two decades, I'm aware of just how important movement and food are to health and well-being. If you've ever tried to make sense of why you know what to do, but struggle to actually do it consistently in the midst of your busy life, this book is for you.

You are not alone. The *what to do* is really the tip of the iceberg when it comes to embodying the healthiest version of yourself.

The real reasons why you're not doing those things—and how to overcome them—is what this book is really about.

You can live the life of your dreams, and it starts with taking control of your health.

Let's dive in!

PART 1

CHAPTER 1

WHY WE'RE HERE

"I know what to do, I'm just not doing it," sighed the frustrated woman on the other end of the phone. I could hear the *Cocomelon* in the background and sensed Monica's anxiety that the tunes wouldn't keep her toddler entertained for our whole conversation, a concern I experienced on a near-daily basis.

That single statement, "I know what to do, I'm just not doing it," is one I've heard uttered by nearly all of the hundreds of women I've talked to about losing weight over the last two decades.

I flashed back to my mid-20s, early in my career as a personal trainer and nutrition coach, well-versed in exercise and nutrition sciences, technically knowing what to do, yet struggling to consistently apply that knowledge to my own life and actually do it!

I didn't yet understand the psychology of behavior change or how to translate textbook knowledge to the real world, which left me stuck in my own miserable cycles of deprivation and restriction, desperate to find a way out.

Take, for example, my weekly fro-yo cheat meal.

Every week, I would fantasize about the oversized concoction I would make on Sunday to reward myself for sticking to all my made-up food rules, eating only low-calorie foods, and restricting myself (aka being "good") all week.

Every week, I'd walk the block and a half from my newly built apartment in Virginia Beach to the local yogurt shop, where I'd fill a large cup to the brim, carefully adding topping after topping. I'd slow-walk over to the high schooler behind the counter and put it on the scale, my mouth watering in anticipation.

After getting over the sticker shock, I'd hurry outside and gobble it up so fast I would barely taste it.

Within minutes, I'd be scraping the bottom and starting the walk of shame back to my apartment, stuffed and guilty for being so "bad."

And yet, the second the door closed behind me, I'd be scouring the cabinets for something else, *anything* else, to eat. My first stop would be any open cereal boxes that I could polish off without the guilt of knowing I'd eaten the *whole* thing. Then I'd go for the chips, crackers, anything crunchy. When I didn't have any temptations on hand (in an effort to prevent this very spiral), I scraped the back of the pantry for the half-eaten bag of shredded coconut left over from my Paleo baking days.

All this because I felt like I'd already blown the day so I thought I might as well keep going. My mindset at the time was, if I kept eating, maybe I would feel so sick and disgusted with myself that I'd never want to do it again.

Except I did. Every week. For months, and after that, less frequently for years.

The food I was eating isn't the important piece of the story. The important part of the story is my restrictive all-or-nothing mentality, my relationship with food, and how I treated myself and my body. And I could tell that the woman on the phone was having similar struggles.

I pulled myself back to my phone conversation. "I'm tired of being in the "tried it all" club," she continued. "I make progress but the weight creeps back on when there is a setback and I've yo-yoed a thousand times. I'm exhausted from constantly thinking about food choices and the emotional consequences they have for me. I need something permanent that will help me to make the positive changes I need for myself, my life, and my family!"

Monica—like I had been, like *my* mom had been—was tired.

Tired of trying so hard and having so little to show for it.

Tired of sacrificing so much for results that barely lasted.

Tired of feeling like something was wrong with her and like she was just doomed to keep gaining weight until the end of time.

I didn't ask, but I felt sure Monica's own mother had likely felt the same way; it's impossible to overestimate the impact our childhood experiences have on us as adults.

Despite vague childhood memories of my mom's Slim Fast shakes and Denise Austin workout tapes, I know my mom must have been very intentional about shielding me from the dark side of dieting: the pain of getting dressed but feeling like nothing she owned looked good, the toll it was taking on her confidence to feel like she couldn't figure it out, the emotional turmoil of getting complimented on her most recent loss, only to gain the weight back shortly after.

She worked hard to make sure her issues didn't become mine, and though I developed plenty of my own body-image and food-related issues, my main memories of her (I lost her to cancer in my early 20s) are those of kindness, compassion, and the belief that external beauty is second to who we are on the inside.

I know many women aren't as fortunate, and their childhood memories are riddled with attending Weight Watchers meetings in dingy church basements or standing in the full-length mirror next to their moms, who picked apart everything they didn't like about their bodies. An informal poll I conducted in my Facebook group, Live Diet-Free, suggests many women have been dieting since early adolescence, with many starting as young as 8.

A shocking 69.4% of American women and 35.4% of American children[1] (age 2-19) are overweight or obese, despite 56.4% of women[2] trying to lose weight in the last 12 months! This doesn't even take into account the droves of women who have given up trying to lose weight because their efforts feel futile.

Maybe you feel like *losing* weight is the easy part, but keeping it off is the struggle. If so, you're not alone: the majority of people who successfully get weight off in the first place end up gaining it back within a handful of years. A meta-analysis of 29 long-term weight loss studies shows the abysmal reality of weight maintenance: more than half of lost weight was regained within two years, and by five years more than 80% of lost weight was regained[3].

---

[1] https://www.niddk.nih.gov/health-information/health-statistics/overweight-obesity
[2] https://www.cdc.gov/nchs/products/databriefs/db313.htm
[3] https://www.ncbi.nlm.nih.gov/pmc/articles/PMC5764193/

To me, these statistics make it blatantly obvious that this skinny-at-any-cost, hate-yourself-thin attitude isn't just unhealthy; it doesn't work!

To be clear, there is *nothing* wrong with having a weight-loss goal if you want one, and this *doesn't* mean you should give up on losing weight if that's what you want. It's just important to know that it's going to take a different approach if you want to be among the minority of women who successfully lose weight and keep it off.

What it does mean is taking a comprehensive, lifestyle-based approach, and knowing that the external habits that support weight loss that lasts will feel much easier when you also do the inner work. That looks like matching your identity to your values and getting clear on the vision you have for your future and how losing weight will get you one step closer to making that your reality.

Taking control of your health can change everything for you, and this book will teach you exactly how.

The Gone For Good formula I'm teaching you in this book will help you lose weight—without sacrificing your health or sanity in the process—*and* be able to keep it off long term. The 3 components, learning and mastering the exercise & nutrition "Big Rocks" (the handful of key behaviors that generate the majority of results), surrounding yourself with comprehensive support, and developing compassionate ownership, will allow you to maintain a healthy and happy weight without obsession or overwhelm.

I'll be going into the "Big Rocks" in Part 2, but I think explaining where the term originated will help you throughout the book. It's really easy to get caught up in trying to do and change *everything* in an effort to lose weight. Think of each of those things (like a fasting window, restricting carbs, burning 500 calories per treadmill workout, etc.) like pebbles or grains of sand you're dropping into an empty jar. Not only will it take a really long time and a lot of energy to fill it up that way, but when you try to put in a bigger rock, there won't be room!

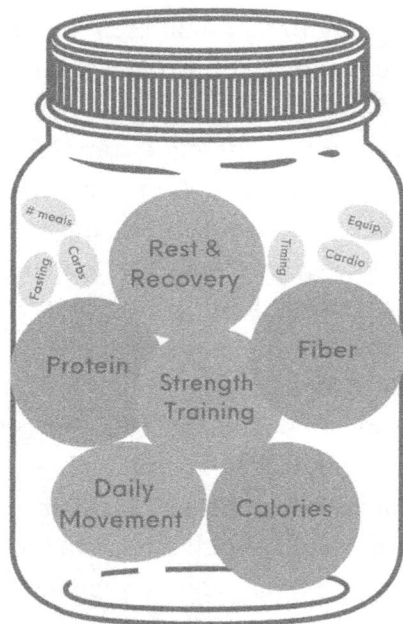

The "Big Rocks" approach you'll learn in this book allows you to fill your jar efficiently by prioritizing the most impactful behaviors that generate the majority of your results.. Once you've done that, if you *want* to spend additional time and energy on the smaller "pebbles" or sand, you can (they'll "fit in the jar").

I created this formula after spending the better part of the last two decades in pursuit of as much information as I could learn about exercise, nutrition, psychology, behavior modification, and lifestyle change. I'm obsessed with learning, to improve my *own* life, my clients' lives, and now yours.

I'm a certified personal trainer, nutrition coach, sports nutritionist, life, health, and weight-loss coach, and I've worked full-time in the fitness & health industry since I graduated from Boston University in 2006 with a degree in Exercise Science. Since then, I have worked in all sorts of settings, from commercial gym chains to corporate wellness, boutique fitness, and community recreation centers before opening the virtual doors to my online business, EA Coaching. I've had the opportunity to support thousands of women in the successful pursuit of their weight-loss and health goals.

I have not always enjoyed working out and eating salads, and if you think I've never had any mental baggage around food—you'd be wrong.

As you probably gathered from my fro-yo story, my own health, weight, and body-image journey has not been without its ups and downs. I've experienced firsthand the shame of needing to buy bigger clothes because none of mine fit after gaining a lot of weight. I know the shame of eating thousands of calories in the grocery store parking lot before throwing away the evidence and trying to pretend it didn't happen. **I know the frustration of knowing what to do to live a healthier and happier lifestyle—but not doing it!**

Much of my pursuit of knowledge has been for my own good. I needed to figure out how to stop bingeing at night, restricting foods all week, and going off the rails on weekends. I needed to learn how to cope with my emotions instead of turning to food. I needed to learn how to exercise for my health, not to burn calories or punish myself.

Now I have a body I love, a healthy relationship with food and exercise, and the confidence to know these will always be constants in my life, but it took me years of trial-and-error to get here.

Thinking about what would have helped my mom get off the weight-loss roller coaster has helped shape my coaching style and methodologies.

I knew that the shakes and VHS tapes (that are probably still in a box somewhere in my childhood house) didn't work—and never would. She, like any busy mom, got tired of liquid meals and fell out of the workout habit when taking care of me, overseeing the local homeless teen shelter, or attending rallies for important causes monopolized all her time.

I understood the complexity of challenges pulling her back into old habits after each loss. I knew that she wasn't hopeless and *could* have found long-term success and that she deserved empathy in the process. I can't help but wonder what might have been different if she'd had the Gone For Good formula.

And so, everything I do to help other women lose weight for good is also for her.

The formula I'm sharing has proven successful on hundreds of busy moms who want to be healthy, happy, and confident—and maybe even lose weight, once and for all.

Throughout the book, I'll share more with you about my own struggles and how I overcame them. I'll also introduce you to several clients, or amalgamations of clients, who will help you see yourself and how the information applies to you.

In Part 1, we're going to talk about four reasons why lasting weight loss has been so evasive thus far:

- Diets encourage restriction, deprivation, and an all-or-nothing mentality.

- Diets are impersonal, isolating, and rely on negativity to fuel surface-level change.

- The modern world is tailored to make it hard to maintain a healthy weight.

- Blame culture makes it easy to shirk responsibility.

You will see that your past "failures" do not mean there's something wrong with you or that you're "doomed to be fat forever." Understanding these four issues will illuminate a clear path forward, this time *avoiding* the pitfalls that claim most dieters.

I'll then share with you the qualities I've found are essential for successfully reaching weight-loss goals, or any goals for that matter. The 3 Cs of Success—Consistency, Commitment, and Confidence—are not characteristics you either have or not, but they are skills you can hone once you realize how important they are (and I'll show you how).

In Part 2, I'm breaking down my game-changing Gone For Good formula (named after my signature coaching program) and showing you exactly what you need in order to lose weight one more time—this time for good.

You'll learn the six exercise and nutrition "Big Rock" habits that will eliminate the overwhelm of starting a weight loss program (*again*) and help you see better results with more flexibility and freedom than ever before. You'll learn how to surround yourself with the kind of comprehensive support that you need (and *deserve*) in order to be in the minority of people who successfully keep the weight off. And lastly, you'll learn how taking compassionate ownership of your results is the key to developing the unwavering confidence that you can handle whatever obstacles and setbacks life throws your way—without gaining the weight back.

In part 3, I'm giving you everything you need to implement the Gone For Good formula in a way that makes sense for *you*, from how to set better goals that don't eventually end up working against you, to developing the cornerstone habit of weekly "life admin" so you're never again scrambling and hoping for the best. You'll also be filling up your Obstacle Toolbox with whatever tools it is YOU need in order to develop the steadfast confidence of a woman who just *knows* she is ready for any challenge she'll face in the future—without reverting back to old habits and regaining all the weight.

In addition, I've compiled helpful resources for you in an exclusive book portal (www.estheravant.com/book-portal-signup), just for purchasing this book and making a commitment to reaching your health and weight-loss goals in a way that lasts. In it you'll find worksheets with all the journaling prompts you'll find throughout this book, a 30-day strength training program with demo videos, workout tracker, calorie calculator, and more.

My hope for you is that you'll not passively read the beginning of this book and then let it collect dust on your nightstand while you go back to doom scrolling. That you'll not just absorb the contents but you'll *implement* the lessons into your life and use this as an opportunity to try to lose weight again, this time **armed with everything you need to be successful.**

I know that if you do, the next few months will be incredibly transformative for you, mentally, physically, and emotionally.

I want to remind you, again, that you don't *have* to want to lose weight. While the specifics may differ, the Gone For Good formula of "Big Rock" habits plus a robust support system plus taking compassionate ownership of the process, is applicable to pretty much any health or lifestyle goal you may want to pursue.

If you *do* want to lose weight, this book will help you do it more successfully and help you get results you're confident can last a lifetime.

This isn't another diet book filled with cabbage soup recipes and lightweight exercises for your "bat wings" (aka upper arm skin that society has taught us to feel shame about—but why?! It's just skin that wobbles thanks to gravity!) I know you don't want another restrictive diet that works until you decide to eat something besides roughage. You don't want to know what will only work for a 20-something with no kids or responsibilities monopolizing every minute of her day.

This book isn't just one I wish I had 10 years ago; it's one I wish my mom had when *she* was struggling with her weight. This book will help remind you that you are a worthy human being deserving of love and respect *regardless* of your size and *also*, how to lose weight and prioritize your health (and yourself) in a compassionate way that will get you lasting results.

Think about the ripple effect you could have on the world, just by deciding to reach your weight loss goal in a way that leaves you feeling healthy, happy, confident, and empowered that you can tackle any goal you want.

The lives of an entire generation of kids—daughters, especially—will be improved by having moms who break their family's generational patterns of negative body image, yo-yo dieting, and unhealthy lifestyle.

Imagine the impact women, in general—and *you*, specifically—could have on our families, communities, and the world if we were mentally and physically stronger and healthier, if we believed in ourselves instead of feeling bogged down by negative self-talk, if we pursued our passions instead of constantly obsessing about food and our bodies.

I wrote this book because I don't want you to spend another day not getting the most out of your life because you don't believe in yourself, aren't happy, or in good enough health to pursue your passions. I *know* that the person you become while prioritizing yourself and your health from a place of love can be the catalyst for incredible transformation.

I know that once you get a taste of setting a goal, laying out a plan, **following through** on it, and seeing that you can do it, you'll be unstoppable. This is the same formula I've used in my own life, and the confidence it has given me has helped me take the leap of faith to quit my job to start my own thriving business, start a podcast that has reached thousands of women, and finally write the book you're currently holding in your hands.

I can't wait to see how YOU choose to get more out of life once you're living with health, happiness, and confidence.

Are you ready? Let's do this!

CHAPTER 2

WHY MOST DIETS FAIL
(IT'S NOT YOU, IT'S THEM)

A ccording to data by Marketdata Enterprises, Americans spend more than $60 billion per year on weight-loss products and services.[4] And yet, the overwhelming majority of Americans who *do* lose weight will gain it back within a handful of years (if not months).

What most people are doing to lose weight is not working when it comes to long-term success.

Why not?

ISSUE 1: Diets encourage restriction, deprivation, and an all-or-nothing mentality.

My client Stacy is the perfect example of this first reason. Stacy's parents both died young, primarily from diseases related to the unhealthy lifestyles they lived for decades. Now

---

[4] https://money.usnews.com/money/personal-finance/articles/2013/01/02/the-heavy-price-of-losing-weight

the mom of a teenager not much younger than she was when they passed, she was desperate to not follow in their footsteps.

She was consistently working out at Orangetheory but regularly felt unfit and like she was going to pass out.

She had "success" with really restrictive programs that required her to eat tiny, cardboard-like, packaged "meals" that she eventually couldn't stomach anymore, but the results were always short-lived. As soon as she started seeing some movement on the scale, she'd feel like she could ease up and go back to eating dinner with her family, and the weight would creep back on.

She pursued similar diet after similar diet, gaining and losing the same 30 pounds, each time blaming her lack of motivation for why she couldn't maintain.

Most dieters approach weight loss with a short-term mentality. You want to fit into a bridesmaid's dress that isn't doing even your thinnest friend any favors. You know you're going to see an ex at an event and want to look good so he knows you're thriving without him. You want to see a certain weight on the scale before a milestone birthday to reaffirm that you're not over the hill.

You trick yourself into thinking you're doing this diet as a "kickstart," and then you'll figure out a healthy way to maintain it once you get there.

But when you finish a restrictive program, all you can think about is how exhausted you are from the gym beatdowns and all the food you're missing because it's been deemed "off-limits" on some list.

You're tired of being "good," so you tell yourself you deserve a break and give yourself the weekend to sleep in and have all the foods you've been missing, and then you'll stick as close to the program as you can after that.

Except that weekend pause spills over into the next week. And the next. And before you know it, it's been weeks or months, and you've lost all that progress for which you've sacrificed so much.

You blame your lack of discipline or willpower and become even more convinced that a strict program with black-and-white rules is the only option for you.

As a perfectionist and people pleaser, it's easy for you to get pulled back into the trap of believing that you're just not good enough. Instead of looking inward and really assessing the gaps in your current skills and knowledge that you'll need to address to make lasting change, you convince yourself that you *need* the rules, to be told exactly what to do, the clear-cut directions about how to do it "right," and someone to berate you if you're less than perfect.

This mentality and the programs that foster them will ALWAYS keep you stuck on the weight-loss rollercoaster!

ISSUE 2: Diets are impersonal, isolating, and reliant on negativity to fuel surface-level change.

Unlike Stacy, my client Jessica knew she couldn't do another restrictive diet, so she hired a popular online macro coach to calculate her targets and hold her accountable with weekly check-ins.

She was convinced this would be the thing. Flexibility and accountability. Exactly what she needed.

Except when she received her "custom" macro targets, they were just a bunch of numbers in a Google Doc with impersonal, copied-and-pasted instructions on how to download a tracking app and enter the targets.

Jessica felt like she was reading a foreign language. She didn't know what any of it meant, and when she asked for help in the client Facebook group, she got hundreds of responses that made her feel stupid and isolated for not knowing the simplest things.

Already her own toughest critic, this sent her into a shame spiral. She was used to being good at things and had expected this to be the same. She wasn't just falling short of her own incredibly high expectations; she was tearing into herself. She'd be mortified if anyone heard the things she was saying to herself, but she really felt like if she couldn't figure this out, she was obviously doomed to be a fat and miserable failure for the rest of her life. She'd probably end up homeless and alone and all because she couldn't figure out this stupid macros thing!

Despite it being incredibly hard for her to reach out for help in the first place, she'd already spent the money, so she was committed to making the most of it. When it came time to do her first check-in with her coach, she poured her heart out about how defeated she was feeling and how she really needed some more guidance and support.

When she finally got a response several days later, she felt even worse. Although the response was so generic and impersonal that she wasn't sure if her coach had even read her message, it just exacerbated how she was feeling by stressing that she just needed to try harder and be more disciplined.

The coach didn't respond with empathy or understanding, meet Jessica where she was, or use it as an opportunity to help her learn how to treat herself with compassion and to reframe her "failures" as opportunities to learn and grow. So Jessica spiraled deeper and deeper into self-hatred and defeat.

By a few weeks in, she had given up, but no one seemed to notice. When she needed help the most, she felt like nothing more than a number.

Most weight-loss programs are focused on surface-level change, supplying you with the "WHAT to do" but leaving you high and dry when it comes to figuring out HOW to make those things work with *your* lifestyle.

Those programs might look good on paper, but they're not designed to help you actually implement them in the midst of shuttling kids to and from activities, putting the final touches on a work presentation, and trying to get to the bottom of the endless pile of laundry.

They don't include the support you need to look at the demands on your time, the mental load you're constantly under, your family and work obligations, and what to do when life throws you curveballs.

When I teach you the exercise & nutrition "Big Rock" habits that generate the majority of your results (Chapters 6 & 7), you'll see that while the "WHAT" is important, it's also pretty straightforward.

The difficult part of weight loss that lasts isn't knowing *what* to do. The most difficult part is addressing all the other elements that make it hard to do those things on a consistent enough basis that you see results, they feel habitual, and you can maintain them long term.

The bulk of this work is beneath the surface, mindset- and lifestyle-related, and totally unaddressed by most programs.

Without education, guidance, flexibility, connection, and empathic accountability, it's incredibly hard to make lasting changes. Again, this leaves you blaming yourself for your lack of follow-through and jumping from program to program in hopes that the next one will somehow provide you what you need.

ISSUE 3: The modern world is tailored to make it hard to maintain a healthy weight.

This was never more apparent to me than after returning from Europe a few months ago.

Headphones in hand, podcast queued up, I stepped out of the resort in Gulf Shores, Alabama, ready to get my walk on. Only to realize there was no wide, wooden boardwalk to stroll along while I got caught up on the latest true crime drama. On the other side of the resort: four lanes of fast-moving traffic with a narrow shoulder and no sidewalks.

Having just moved back to the U.S. after three years in Europe, this surprised me. I was used to walking, whether on city streets or the endless miles of trails traversing all the small towns.

The surprise continued when I found myself at the local Wal-Mart, where I must have looked like an alien dropped in from outer space as I snapped pictures of two dozen marshmallow varieties to send to my husband with a ☺ emoji.

It was my first time in an American grocery store in three years, and I was walking up and down the aisles with my mouth agape at all the hundreds of brightly colored snack and dessert options.

Since we'd landed back in the U.S. a week prior, I had been shocked by the excess I was seeing, well, everywhere.

Restaurants serving outrageously sized portions of delicious, salty, sugary, fatty goodness.

400-calorie drinks.

900-calorie salads.

1,200-calorie appetizers.

2,000-calorie entrees and desserts.

Every intersection had more fast food restaurants than corners. Even the FedEx I popped into to return an Amazon package had a brightly colored candy display and soda cooler near the checkout.

With almost 70% of American women being overweight or obese, I can't write this book and not mention how much modern society is contributing to the challenge of losing weight.

People who reach and maintain a healthy weight are in the minority. The odds are stacked against you. Technology has made it easier than ever to move less and eat more. You can work from home, and any time we turn on the TV or open social media, you're bombarded with food and drinks you can order directly from your phone.

Your social life often revolves around eating and drinking to excess, although it doesn't feel excessive because it's what everyone else is doing. Most people's habits are the exact opposite of the ones that will make lasting weight loss possible, and the status quo bias (people's preference for keeping things the way they are) is strong. It's much harder to turn down another round of cocktails or decline dessert when it's what everyone else is doing and something you've normally done.

Wanting to lose weight isn't unusual (see $60-billion industry), but doing so in a way that will last and you're not jumping on the latest diet de jour makes you an outlier among your peers.

Becoming part of the minority requires consistently behaving differently. Going against said status quo, standing out, being "weird"—like brown-bagging it at lunch instead of going out, or being the one mom at the playground doing push-ups on a bench. And not just on occasion, but doing those things over and over and over again until they become the norm for you, all while the constant barrage of temptations and pressure to conform continue. Don't be discouraged, though. It's entirely possible for you when you develop things like compassionate ownership and finding like-minded people (which I cover later in this book).

ISSUE 4: Blame culture makes it easy to shirk responsibility.

Several years ago, I saw this post in a Facebook group:

> "Well, I cried this morning. I need to lose this weight (60+ pounds). I started riding my Peloton, again. I'm eating better. I cut back on wine to just weekends. I'm not snacking nearly as much. I feel like I've been working SO hard this month and I GAINED a pound. I cried. The first time I ever cried about my weight. It's so discouraging to work at it only to see the numbers go up. Honestly, it makes me want to just give up. It doesn't feel possible. What am I doing wrong?"

The responses came flying in. Within an hour of this post, over 200 women with good intention had chimed in with their two cents. It was clear to me that nearly everyone was trying to find something to blame:

"Get a thyroid panel."

"Wear a continuous glucose monitor."

"Have your hormones checked."

"You probably don't have the genetics to lose weight."

"You probably have a slow metabolism."

"I gained 50 pounds with menopause."

"Get a prescription for phentermine."

"Maybe you have PCOS."

I'm not saying these aren't valid concerns that may make losing weight feel extra challenging. Some people do have thyroid or autoimmune issues that result in a reduced basal metabolic rate. Hormonal fluctuations or imbalances can have a cascade effect that impacts hunger and satiety, fat storage, and more. Sometimes prescription medications are helpful.

If you have concerns about your health, please see your doctor for regular check-ups, blood work, and to communicate those concerns. If you're not feeling heard or understood, advocate for yourself and, if necessary, find a practitioner who listens to and supports you and feels like an ally.

In my experience, I've found that challenges like these affect a small minority of women and are just that: challenges. Not insurmountable roadblocks.

Medical issues aside, you can find dozens of excuses for why your situation isn't your fault. It's your kids, or their ages, or how many you have. It's your naturally skinny husband who doesn't have to worry about what he eats. It's that your company provides catered lunches you're expected to eat, and clients show their appreciation with food that you're powerless to resist. It's your travel schedule and how impossible it is to make good choices at restaurants. It's your active social life and not wanting everyone to think you're pregnant if you choose not to drink.

These are all factors in your lifestyle that need addressing (or reframing), but the time you spend focusing on these problems (real or imagined) is time not spent on brainstorming and testing the possible solutions to them.

Although you can't control everything, there is a lot you can, and the belief that results are outside your control is defeating and downright dangerous.

Taking ownership of your health and approaching weight loss with a comprehensive, lifestyle-based approach will help you lose weight, keep it off, and improve nearly everything in your life.

Losing weight isn't about fat-blasting workouts, maximizing how many calories you burn on your Peloton, superfoods, ACV shots—any of that.

It's about developing self-awareness, creating the identity of someone who already *is* maintaining a healthy weight, and putting in the work to hone the mindset, skills, and tools that will help you become her.

It IS possible, and doing so will not just help you take control of your health but can also be the catalyst for incredible lifestyle transformation.

I'll show you how in the upcoming chapters, starting with developing the 3 Cs of Success: consistency, commitment, and confidence.

CHAPTER 3

THE 3 CS OF SUCCESS
(OR LACK THEREOF)

"That's a twelve."

Coach Meg, head coach in my Gone For Good program, had asked Kelly to rate—on a scale of 1-10—how important her weight-loss goal was and how committed she was to putting in the work to make it her reality. It's something we ask every woman who applies to work with us.

Most say they're an eight or a nine; losing weight is really important to them, but they have this wedge of doubt that they can actually do it, so they're scared to say they're a ten. While that uncertainty is normal and understandable, it's also easy to let self-doubt takeover and sabotage their efforts before they've even gotten started.

Kelly's unwavering commitment, one of the 3 Cs of Success, right from the start was a sign that she was going to reach her weight-loss—and any other—goal.

Kelly tried for years to get pregnant. All the struggle and sacrifice was worth it for her beautiful three-year-old daughter, Mila, who was the light of her life. But fertility treatments had taken a toll on Kelly's body, and a couple years into motherhood, she felt like she hit rock bottom, heavier now than when she'd given birth and getting winded just bringing the laundry up the stairs.

In the past, that meant hopping back on the Optavia (or other, similar) bandwagon. (Although there may be women who found success with programs like these, they never worked for her long term). But this time had to be different. She knew she had to focus on deeper work, not just starve herself on packaged foods for a few months.

She didn't want her daughter to see her like that—or this. She wanted to lead by example and show Mila what it means to be strong and healthy and confident. And she wasn't feeling any of those things.

Kelly knew raising her daughter was going to require her to put herself out there—to do life—more. But instead of looking forward to her Mila being old enough to experience Disney for the first time, she was nervous. Nervous about being able to fit into the rides, nervous about being able to be on her feet for so long, nervous about what she could wear that would hide her insecurities but not stifle her in the Florida summer heat.

Kelly knew she couldn't do it alone. She had a tendency to self-sabotage, to give up when results didn't come as quickly or as easily as she'd like.

This time she was going to do things differently. Instead of going back to the familiar siren call of something drastic and restrictive, she was ready to learn another way. A way that would last.

In addition to commitment, Kelly also displayed the two other attributes I've seen in my most successful clients over the last two decades: consistency and confidence. She's now lost nearly 90 pounds, dropped numerous clothing sizes, has gotten crazy strong, and continues to set a positive example for Mila every single day.

Don't worry if you don't feel like you're particularly strong at any of these 3 Cs. You already have these qualities within you, and the Gone For Good formula I will teach you in Part 2 will help you develop them into your superpowers.

Consistency, commitment, and confidence will help you lose weight, but the benefits don't stop there. They'll also help you lead a healthy lifestyle, build a body you love, enjoy your life more, and pursue whatever lights you up. Taking a health-first approach is the catalyst for achieving *any* goal you want.

Think of how much more enjoyable life would be if you weren't preoccupied with how you look or how your clothes fit.

Think of how much more energy you'd have to give to the people you love or causes you care about if you weren't toiling away on the treadmill trying to burn as many calories as possible.

Think of how much more productive, creative, or ambitious you'd be if you weren't obsessing over food or your body.

Think of how much more successful you'd be at losing weight if you were making changes to your lifestyle from a place of love and compassion that supported your health and happiness instead of trying to hate yourself skinny.

Everything in your life is better when you make your health and happiness a top priority in your life.

Losing and keeping off weight is **no** different from reaching any other goal. It might *feel* different because you haven't successfully done it (yet), but if you've accomplished any other meaningful goal in your life, you already have the consistency, commitment, and confidence it takes to be successful at losing weight and keeping it off.

Think about graduating from high school or college. That may have been a long, arduous process, but you did it. How?

By showing up more often than not.

Doing the homework, writing the papers, taking the exams.

By **really** wanting the outcome of graduating, whether to appease your parents, set yourself up for the career of your dreams, or any other number of reasons.

You had moments (weeks/months) of frustration when it sucked and felt hard and you didn't want to do it. But the outcome was important enough to you that you stuck it out.

While a diploma or degree is a short-term goal, the skills you develop in the process of achieving it provide the foundation for a lifetime of other accomplishments, just like *losing* weight, done the Gone For Good way, provides the foundation for a lifetime of keeping it off.

Even if you haven't accomplished a big goal in the past, you can still be successful at losing weight and whatever other goals you set because the 3 Cs are not natural abilities or inherent personality traits but, instead, skills you can develop.

Stanford psychologist Carol Dweck is known for her work on motivation and mindset and is the author of *Mindset: The New Psychology of Success*. In her work, she has coined the term "growth mindset," the definition of which I've paraphrased below:

Growth Mindset: Belief that basic abilities *can be developed* through dedication and hard work. You may start with certain natural talents or tendencies, but you are capable of learning, developing, and changing who you are and what you know how to do, even if it's not easy at first.

While reading this book, I want you to try on a growth mindset and believe that you are someone who is capable of learning new things and developing new skills. No longer will you just accept the status quo, believing (incorrectly) that you just have to accept the hand you were dealt, and if that means being stuck in a body you're not comfortable in, lacking energy, being irritable with the people you love the most, staying at a job that's not fulfilling, and generally just not getting the most out of life, so be it. The Gone For Good formula will help you develop the consistency, commitment, and confidence to succeed at losing weight and any goal.

Consistency means showing up day in and day out and engaging in the behaviors that make reaching your weight loss goal more likely (the exercise and nutrition "Big Rocks" we'll cover in chapters 7 and 8). If you go through spurts where you're "on" and prioritizing your weight loss but follow them by periods of being "off" and backsliding into old habits, your consistency is lacking.

Commitment means staying focused on what you want long term in the face of temptations and in spite of periods of low motivation or enthusiasm. If you find yourself derailed by small inconveniences or giving up when the going gets tough, your commitment may be lacking.

Confidence means believing that it's possible for you to learn and do what it takes to reach your weight-loss goal—and keep it off this time. If you find yourself making excuses to justify not starting in the first place or not making your best effort once you do, your confidence may be lacking. Sometimes a lack of confidence is at the root of your lack of consistency or commitment.

Embodying the 3Cs will empower you to know that you have what it takes to lose weight and keep it off. Once you see that all obstacles between you and the weight you want to lose fall under one of the categories of consistency, commitment, or confidence, the path toward a solution becomes that much clearer.

A lack of consistency may be due to trying to do too much at once and spreading yourself too thin, or it may be that you don't have the support and guidance you need.

A lack of commitment may be because you haven't taken the time to scratch beneath the surface and figure out why your goal really matters, or it may be because you're not in the habit of taking ownership of your results.

A lack of confidence may be because you don't believe in yourself, and you're not surrounding yourself with people who help you see your potential. Or it may be that you haven't taken on the identity of a healthy, fit person and, therefore, have trouble showing up as her.

It's important to note that all 3Cs are intertwined, rather than sequential.

A lack of commitment or consistency may boil down to a lack of confidence, but commitment and consistency can help *build* confidence. Consistency helps build commitment and commitment yields consistency.

The 3Cs are not inherent traits that you either have or don't. They're all skills/tools that you can work on building, as we'll dive into in the next few chapters.

You are worthy and deserving of the time and attention it takes to identify the gaps in your skillset and then do the work to develop those areas.

Being consistent, committed, and confident—and the *tools* you develop to exemplify those qualities, day in and day out—aren't just going to help you lose weight and improve your health; they're going to benefit you in literally *every* aspect of your life.

That's what taking a health-first approach will do for you.

The only way to live your best, happiest, most fulfilling life is if you are *also* living your *healthiest* life. It **has** to start with health. *Everything* is impacted by your health.

If you struggle with any (or all) of the 3 Cs, that's normal and you're in good company: most women do. It's not a sign that you're hopeless or there's something wrong with you.

You might want to roll your eyes at me, but I want you to start with some journaling. I know, I know. You might not want to. I didn't, either, until I saw just how powerful a tool journaling can be. So I encourage you to give it a shot. I recommend you follow the prompts from each chapter before moving on to the next.

In addition to journaling prompts, I'm also going to offer other simple tools in each chapter that, when used consistently, will have a big impact on developing the 3Cs, like building out your own personal consistency trackers for the behaviors that matter most to you, getting to the root of why your goal really matters, and engaging in exercises for pulling all the self-doubt out of the darkest corners of your brain.

In the meantime, let's start with these:

Journaling Prompts

Which of the 3Cs (consistency, commitment, confidence) do you think is your biggest area for potential improvement? What makes you think that?

Do you consider any of the 3Cs to be a strength for you? Why or why not?

How will reaching your weight loss goal help you get more out of life?

What cause or movement are you passionate about that you'd be more fully able to pursue if you had the 3Cs and weren't preoccupied with your weight/body/health?

CHAPTER 4

CONSISTENCY

When I was 16, fresh driver's license in hand, I spent every weekday after school driving myself 60 minutes round trip along the back roads of midcoast Maine to the local YMCA after school. I don't know what prompted me to *start* going in the first place (probably boys), and I don't really know why I *kept* going at first (probably boys), but I do know that eventually, after showing up enough, I started to see and feel the results. I started liking how I looked, I started getting more attention from boys, and I started developing a reputation as The Girl Who Went To The Gym After School. That became my identity.

There were days when the winter darkness combined with the heat in my old Volvo made getting out of the car much like getting out of a cozy bed when the alarm goes off at the crack of dawn—the last thing I wanted to do. Sometimes I'd take a cat nap in the parking lot before going in, only getting changed after warming my clothes up with the hair dryer in the locker room.

I knew I'd feel great after finishing my workout, so on the hard days when I just wanted to go home and curl up under blankets, I'd play games with myself:

"All you have to do is scan in."

"Just go down to the locker room."

"See if there are any cute boys playing basketball."

"Get yourself dressed."

"Do five minutes on the elliptical."

Eventually, I would end up doing everything I'd planned on: a short cardio warm-up, a few rounds on the Nautilus circuit, and some extra time on the Stairmaster.

Fast forward a couple of years to my freshman year of college, and I got a taste of the other side of consistency, aka *in*consistency.

Totally over my head with a demanding schedule full of science classes that my small high school hadn't prepared me for and with no one who knew me as The Girl Who Went To The Gym After School, I only worked out a handful of times.

My sophomore year, Boston University built a state-of-the-art fitness center, but freshman year, the only option was an old dingy basement where I would occasionally bring flash cards while I rode the elliptical.

I didn't know what time the cute boys went to help me get into the habit of going consistently, plus I had an ever-growing list of sciency things I didn't understand and needed to learn ASAP.

Between my abysmal gym attendance, unlimited options at the dining hall, all the beer I was drinking, and the pineapple & olive pizza my roommate and I ordered on the regular after getting stoned, I gained over 35 pounds and even outgrew what I derogatorily called my "fat pants" just months later.

Consistency works both ways. I had reaped the benefits of consistently exercising and eating well, and now I was paying the consequences of doing neither. I didn't know it at the time, but I was approaching health and fitness with an all-or-nothing mentality, one of the biggest threats to consistency.

Threat #1 To Health Consistency: All-Or-Nothing Approach

My client Saki was on top of the world. She'd lost 70 pounds on her own and was feeling amazing. She was a fixture in Facebook groups related to her workout program and her 453-day streak was the envy of many.

She was clocking upward of two hours working out every morning: her "therapy."

She wouldn't stop until she'd burned 1,000 calories and meticulously tracked everything that entered her mouth. Not that that was really necessary anymore, since she'd been eating the exact same meals and snacks for well over a year.

Her consistency during the pandemic was admirable. She'd really taken advantage of having nowhere to be and nothing to do. Losing weight had become her top priority.

Except now the world was starting to open up, and Saki was terrified. How could she go back to traveling for work when that would mean having to eat out with other people?! How would she burn enough calories if she didn't have two hours to work out in the morning?

When a time zone debacle resulted in the loss of her Apple Watch streak one day in June, Saki—and her perfect routine—crumbled.

After missing a day of working out, she couldn't bring herself to do the next day. What did it matter? She was already starting over at zero.

Without her massive morning calorie burn, she was scared to eat her normal breakfast of oatmeal with a side of one hard-boiled egg—or eat at all. But by the time eight p.m. rolled around, she was so hungry that she couldn't stop herself from eating everything in sight, including all the "forbidden foods" she'd sworn off over a year ago.

Day after day was the same. She just couldn't pull herself together.

When her scale showed that she was up a couple of pounds, she had visions of regaining all 70 pounds she'd lost, and the spiral continued.

By the time she reached out to me for help, she was up ten pounds and convinced her lack of discipline was the problem.

Consistency is the most tangible of the 3 Cs of success. Your Apple Watch, Fitbit, Peloton, Headspace, MyFitnessPal, and other well-meaning apps are very quick to tell you just how consistent (or inconsistent) you've been.

You're either getting high fives and back pats for your streak, or you're getting gently scolded by some sort of cartoon character in an effort to help you get a few days in a row under your belt. Even without technology, it's pretty easy to tell whether you keep buying lettuce that you throw away at the end of the week or are taking a "pet apple" to and from work every day that you never eat, so it just travels back and forth with you.

Most women are consistently inconsistent. We go through spurts where we're "on" or "good," doing all the things, checking the boxes, feeling proud of ourselves, or, well, none of those things. We're "off," "bad," feeling like crap.

This struggle with consistency stems from an all-too-common phenomenon: having an all-or-nothing mentality, wherein you feel like if you're not making a grandiose effort, overhauling everything at once, then you're not doing enough. You've come to equate misery and suffering with success.

The problem is, it doesn't work. It never has and it never will.

Wanting to go all in makes sense. You're so fed up with how you're feeling that you're *desperate* to take action. The more drastic, the better.

You *want* to suffer. You may even feel like you deserve it.

You may feel like the only way to get out of the hole you're in is to get as far away as possible, seemingly never making the connection between that and why you keep ending up right back in the same place.

Being All In doesn't *feel* like too much at first. You actually feel really good! You're empowered. You feel in control. Proud that you're taking action. Your mid-afternoon crash isn't as crashy and you're not getting as winded taking the laundry upstairs. You start recognizing small changes in how your clothes are fitting, your output on the Peloton, and your mood: all motivating signs that you're on the right track! You're feeling so motivated that continuing to do the things doesn't feel too hard.

In the beginning, when whatever you're doing is new and exciting, it feels like a necessary and worthwhile sacrifice. You're making your goals a priority, often because you've started at a time when it's convenient, like January 1st or eight weeks before a vacation, when the thought of being in a bathing suit motivates you to keep showing up.

But inevitably, life starts to happen. Unlike being a contestant on *The Biggest Loser*, you're not able to escape the reality of your life in order to prioritize your weight-loss goals. You have to juggle it all. And instead of being able to handle life's ups and downs with ease, you feel more like a clown juggling on a unicycle with someone throwing bananas at you until you fall over.

Your new five a.m. cardio and juicing routine may be going just swimmingly . . . until a kid wakes up at three a.m. puking and you're up the rest of the night.

Until a work deadline starts looming and requires late nights.

Until you've cleaned that damn juicer ONE TIME TOO MANY and just want a breakfast that requires teeth to eat and isn't the color of boogers.

Instead of flexing and adjusting, you feel like if you can't maintain all the habits you're trying to build, you might as well not bother with any of them. What good is a daily walk or an earlier bedtime when you can't commit to an hour of cardio and freshly juiced veggies at five a.m.?

The pendulum swings back to "nothing" for a variety of reasons: your new behaviors weren't yet well-established habits that had the longevity to weather a storm, you were spreading yourself too thin by trying to do too much, and you were changing from a place of negativity and hatred for your current body.

Your efforts are best described as spurts. Sometimes you're killing it and have a weeks- or months-long streak. Sometimes all your healthy toys and tools develop a thin layer of dust from lack of use.

Getting out of this all-or-nothing cycle is crucial if you want to develop the consistency you need to reach your weight-loss goals and maintain your results.

Overcoming Your All-Or-Nothing Mentality

Rather than a switch that toggles from 0% to 100%, start thinking about your efforts as radio dials that offer a vast area between all and nothing.

Exercise and nutrition very often get lumped together, as though they operate on the same dial, but they don't. Decoupling them will help you stay out of all-or-nothing territory and see that turning the dial down on one can be an opportunity to turn the dial up on the other.

You already know what zero effort and maximum effort look like; start figuring out the in-between options—for example, doing an abbreviated workout if you're short on time, or getting a side salad instead of fries.

Learning to live in the "messy middle," as one of my clients dubbed it, is the key to showing up more consistently.

Instead of feeling like a failure if you aren't working out seven days a week, look back at the last couple of weeks and set realistic goals based on the other demands on your time and energy.

Take baby steps that you are confident you can do, even on your worst week when life *is* throwing you curveballs, so that you're racking up small wins that build momentum and confidence.

Prove to yourself that you're someone who does what she says she's going to do and develop the mindset of feeling inspired to do a little bit more the following week.

Recognize that *everything* can't be your #1 priority all the time and nothing can be your top priority *all* the time, but your health always needs to be in the top few, so if it's been on the back burner for too long, it's time to reprioritize.

Reminder

You're not going to do *any* one thing every single day. Perfection is unrealistic *and* unnecessary!

Threat #2 To Health Consistency: Flying Under The Radar

Jill *wasn't* trying to do it all. Been there, done that. She was done trying to be perfect and had learned how to give herself grace and accept that life—and her efforts—would have ups and downs.

Instead of obsessing about not missing a day of workouts, she was just getting them in as she was able, usually a couple of times per week.

Instead of following a restrictive diet, she was fasting 16 hours per day, and even though she was technically "allowed" to eat whatever she wanted during her "feeding window," she was confident that she was making pretty healthy choices most of the time.

Mentally, Jill felt way better about her approach than what she'd done in the past, save for one small problem: she wasn't losing any weight. With some coaching, Jill was able to see that maintaining her current weight, rather than gaining steadily as she had each year for the several years prior, was actually a big win! But she still had about 20 pounds she wanted to lose.

She had successfully overcome her all-or-nothing approach to health, but she fell straight into an equally frustrating trap: falling short of the consistency threshold that produces results.

While 100% effort isn't required, losing weight does require a higher level of effort and consistency than maintaining does. I've found that the threshold to transition yourself into weight loss happens around 85% consistency. If you're hitting the exercise and nutrition goals we'll lay out in upcoming chapters about 26 days out of a month, you're very likely to lose weight.

I don't want you to get too hung up on the exact percentage here or to be doing any complicated math equations, just to realize that perfection isn't necessary to lose weight, but a pretty high level of consistency is.

If you're averaging under that, even not by much, you're more likely to maintain your current weight while feeling like you're doing everything right but it's not working. In Chapter 7, I'll provide you with a consistency tracker that will help you see what you're doing well and what areas require more of your attention, but in the meantime, come up with a list of three to five *impactful* behaviors that are important to you and you want to start (or stop) doing.

Some suggestions you could start implementing right away are to get three or more servings of veggies per day, cut out after-dinner snacking, take a morning walk, or get into bed at whatever time allows you to get at least seven hours of sleep. Print a blank calendar and steal some stickers or markers from your kids (or workplace!) and start tracking your consistency with those behaviors ASAP.

One issue to look out for is focusing your energy on habits that aren't actually as impactful as you think. In Jill's case, fasting is a *tool* that can be useful for some women to make being in a caloric deficit feel easier, but it's not a guarantee that she would be eating the right amounts of the right things to see the weight loss she was after. By the end of Chapter 7, you'll be crystal clear on which habits give you the most bang for your buck and which may just be a distraction or energy drain.

If you're doing the "Big Rocks" 85% of the time and you're *still* not losing weight, it's time to look at whether you're going through the motions just to check the boxes, or if you're showing up with the effort of someone who understands and believes that each individual workout and meal choice matters and is an opportunity to get a little bit closer to your weight loss goal.

Reminder

Showing up and showing up to the best of your ability are two different things.

Threat #3 To Health Consistency: Expectation Management

"That's *it!*" Emma yelled into the empty bathroom, seriously considering throwing the scale into the mirror.

Her husband knew enough to give her space on weigh-in days. He was downstairs, waiting to hear whether she came floating down the stairs with glee or stomping down trying to stifle her sobs.

Today? Stomping.

Once again, the number wasn't what Emma wanted to see, despite being consistent all week.

She just didn't understand why, no matter what she did, it felt like she couldn't lose more than a pound or so each week. Not to mention the weeks it was even less or went *up* for some godforsaken reason!

The rest of the weekend could go one of two ways: reverting back to her all-or-nothing mentality that if last week's effort somehow wasn't good enough, she'd need to be even *more* perfect this week . . . or getting a case of the F*ck Its and soothing her emotions with all the food and drinks she'd been denying herself all week, only to start over again on Monday.

Unrealistic expectations—and how we react to our perceived mismatch of effort and progress—are one of the main factors contributing to inconsistency, unnecessary frustration, and lack of weight-loss results.

Many women anchor their weight-loss expectations to completely unrealistic ideals set forth by social media or old shows like *The Biggest Loser*. Never mind that these big weekly drops aren't healthy or sustainable; most women experiencing rapid weight loss will gain it back! I know it would be nice to just get to your weight-loss goal and be done with the whole thing, but your goal is to *keep it off*, which means not being so focused on the quick wins that you lose sight of what matters most: reaching your goal with the ability to—and confidence that you can—stay there, no matter what life throws at you.

Keep in mind that "slow" weight loss isn't *actually* slower when you factor in all the yo-yo-ing most women experience when they approach weight loss in a more drastic and restrictive way.

The initial drops on the scale might be motivating (though keep in mind they're largely water and muscle), but inevitably, most women are going to be unable to maintain that approach for long and are likely to gain it back, often with some additional pounds.

Healthy and sustainable fat loss is generally in the range of .5-1% of your body weight per week, which for most women is in the range of half a pound to two pounds. This is very rarely linear because of how dynamic our bodies are and how easily impacted the scale is by a number of variables.

The thing to ask yourself when this feels so painstakingly slow is: would you rather lose 25-75 pounds this year in a way you know you can keep off? Or 25 pounds this quarter, only to gain back 30 pounds the next quarter, lose it again in Q3, and then finish out the year right back where you started?

Lasting weight loss takes consistent action over long periods of time. Even then, results are still going to come slower than you might like. If your goal is to lose weight and KEEP IT OFF, you will be much more successful accepting this than continuing to try to hack the system.

Determine Your Weight Loss Time Frame

Current Weight: _____

Goal Weight: _____

Total Pounds You Want To Lose: _____

Weeks It Will Take At .5lbs/week (pounds you want to lose TIMES 2): _____

Weeks It Will Take At 2lbs/week (pounds you want to lose DIVIDED by 2): _____

Time Range To Lose Desired Weight: _____ to _____ weeks

Add 2-4 weeks of extra time to this range for life happening (getting sick, going away, getting busy, just reverting back to old habits, etc.).

Adjusted range: _____ to _____ weeks

Although these numbers might be a million times longer than you'd like, it's better to be prepared for the long haul than continue to be frustrated by unrealistic expectations.

Reminder

Your "slow" weight loss isn't really slow if you keep it off instead of gaining it back!

A Word On Motivation

You will not always be motivated. You'll need to keep showing up regardless of how you're feeling, but a lack of motivation from time to time is not a problem.

Part of why building routines and habits is so important for maintaining consistency is because taking action breeds motivation.

There will be times when you just don't want to do the exercise and nutrition "Big Rocks." I call this "the Grind"; it's inevitable and not a cause for concern.

There will be times when you're frustrated by how slowly your results are coming and how hard you're working.

There will be times when your habits and skills still feel clunky and unnatural, like they're taking a lot of energy and seem to be having such a minimal impact on your progress.

There will be times when you can see that you're not where you started but you feel like you still have a long way to go before you get to where you want to be, and it just sucks.

There will be times when your drive is at an all-time low and you really want to throw in the towel.

Quitting during these times will not help you reach your weight-loss goal. "The Grind" is an opportunity to practice adjusting your dials to levels that feel manageable for you to continue to show up and do more than nothing, and to lean on your support system to help you stay consistent regardless of motivation.

While motivation is a feeling, it's also a skill. Believing that YOU are in control of your day-to-day choices and that each individual one contributes to reaching your larger, meaningful goal is crucial to building the skill of intrinsic motivation. (See more in Commitment and Confidence chapters).

Consistency is something you can focus on now, and you'll also notice that developing commitment and confidence makes consistency easier.

Journaling Prompt

Write down all the obstacles that challenge your consistency with taking meaningful action. For each, list at least one solution so you are better prepared with solutions rather than excuses.

Obstacle	Solution

CHAPTER 5

COMMITMENT

"How'd it go?" my now-familiar cabbie asked when I got back into his car.

"I won't find out for six to eight weeks, but I'm pretty sure I failed," I said, feeling defeated. Earlier in the year, I'd committed to getting my personal training certification, and I'd studied every day for the months leading up to test day—today.

A few hours earlier I'd spent the 40-minute ride to the testing center anxiously trying to remember muscle insertion and origin points, and now he was bringing me back to my dorm in the middle of Kenmore Square in Boston.

Successfully getting myself to and from the test felt like the only win of the day. The actual test was anticlimactic since I didn't walk out with a pass or a fail, just a "Thanks for coming. We'll send your results to the address we have on file."

Turns out I *did* pass (and I heard in more like four weeks rather than eight!), but this was our reality less than 20 years ago. We wanted things and we first had to work for them. . . and then we had to wait for them.

Now, instead of walking to the mailbox for a catalog, making the phone call to a sales rep to order, and waiting weeks or months for our delivery, we tap a few buttons on our phones and Amazon will send us nearly anything we want within 24 hours.

We've gotten accustomed to near-instant gratification, so it's no *wonder* that we want our weight loss to come quickly and easily.

Except that the things most worth having still require time, effort, and commitment over longer periods, just like the work it took to prepare for the personal training certification that started to shape my future career.

When it comes to losing weight, focusing on quick results very often means *losing* those results just as quickly, which just further perpetuates the yo-yo cycle. The more successful approach to losing weight—and the one that most women *don't* take—is going about it in a way that will make *maintaining* your progress easier for the rest of your life.

I **don't** mean being more restrictive, working out more, eating less and less, trying to be more perfect, or any of that. I mean actually learning the skills and tools that you need to lose weight for good, live a healthy lifestyle, and change your life.

The real work isn't finding someone to write you a meal plan or treat you like you're in boot camp. Don't get me wrong, the exercise and nutrition stuff matters (we'll get into that in Chapter 7), but the real work isn't just about knowing what to do, it's about figuring out *how* to actually do it consistently and **why** it matters to you! Knowing why it really matters if you lose weight will help you overcome the most common threats to commitment.

Threat #1 To Commitment: Vague and Surface Level Goals

If we were having a conversation and I asked you why you want to lose weight, you might say something like:

"None of my clothes fit. I don't want to buy a bigger size."

"I hate how I look."

"I can't believe I've gotten this big."

"I haven't weighed this much since I was pregnant and my youngest is seven!"

"I felt good at one fifty, so I just want to get back there."

All those reasons to want to lose weight are valid (though I do encourage you to practice self-love and acceptance no matter your size). Seeing a smaller number on the scale feels good, and it's really nice to be able to shop your own closet instead of seeing dollar signs of all the money you've wasted on too-small clothes.

But if the *only* thing driving you is seeing a smaller number on the scale, it's very hard to stay committed when you inevitably go through spells of *not* seeing the scale move, and especially when you reach maintenance and the goal is for that number *not* to change.

I *know* your reasons for wanting to lose weight run deeper than these.

It's not just that you don't feel good at this weight; it's also that you're constantly irritable and snapping at your husband and kids.

It's not just that none of your clothes fit; it's that you feel like no one at work takes you seriously. (I've heard this from many of my clients, and it makes me incredibly sad and frustrated to see how our society treats people of different sizes differently, which isn't right and isn't fair.)

It's not just that you feel like you're turning into your mom; it's seeing the lifestyle-related health complications she's experiencing and fearing them in your future, too.

It's not just that you hate how you look; it's that you miss the fun you used to have when you felt confident in yourself.

It's not just that you're over your pregnancy weight; it's that you see your kids growing up so fast and you fear you won't be healthy or alive long enough to see them grow up, graduate, and have kids of their own.

It's not just that you want to see a number from your past; it's that you miss the person you were, how you felt about yourself, and the way you lived your life back then.

These are the types of compelling reasons that build commitment to your goals and help you stick things out and stay consistent when the going gets tough (and it will).

The more specific you can get with what your goal actually is and why it's important to you, the better, because then you can reverse engineer a plan to get you from where you are to where you want to be. (More on goal-setting in Chapter 9).

"5 Whys" Exercise

You've probably seen, "What's Your WHY?" exercises before, so try not to gloss over it because you "know this already." Understanding what's driving you and why it's important that you lose this weight is crucial for developing the commitment necessary to actually follow through and do it.

List your weight loss goal: _____

Just like when you're having a conversation with a toddler, keep asking yourself, "Why, why, why?"

Why do I want to lose _____ pounds?* _____

Why is that important to me? _____

Why does it matter? _____

Why do I need it? _____

And why is that important? _____

Peeling back the layers like this can produce incredible insights that can deepen your commitment to your goals.

*Note: You can do this exercise with goals unrelated to weight, such as wanting certain clothes to fit or physical things you'd like to be able to do. It's likely that in going through this exercise, you realize that a specific "goal weight" isn't really what you're after so much as more energy, confidence, joy, etc.

Journal Prompts

Spend a few minutes journaling on the following prompts that will help you expand on the insights from the "5 Whys" Exercise and combat the first threat to commitment:

How will reaching your goal change your life?

Who will you become in the process of losing weight?

What's really at the root of your emotional reason for needing to reach your goal?

Why does losing weight really matter to you? What does it represent for you?

Why will it be worth continuing to show up, even when it's hard, inconvenient, you're tired, don't have time, and can think of all the excuses in the book?

Threat #2 to Commitment: Being In The Minority

I've mentioned how dismal the statistics are on long-term weight maintenance. I don't remind you of those to scare you or make you feel defeated, but to prepare you for the fact that having something that most women want but won't achieve requires you to do things that most women don't. To go against the grain. You'll be an outlier, and your choices will put you in the minority a lot of the time. You might feel like a weirdo or like people are judging you.

And they might be.

I've certainly been judged for my commitment to my workouts or my food choices. Many years ago I worked as the fitness manager at a recreation center that held staff potlucks every month or so. I always packed my lunch but attended my first potluck, anyway, in an effort to be a good team player. Just about everyone I spoke to that lunch made some comment along the lines of, "Of *course* you brought your own lunch; that's what you 'healthy people' do," or "You probably can't eat any of this 'bad' stuff, can you?" (gesturing to the row of Crockpots, each holding a different spin on a cheese dip).

I couldn't have cared less what my coworkers were choosing to eat, but just my presence there, eating something besides the buffet options, made them defensive and judgmental toward me.

What I reminded myself of, and what I want you to remember, is that situations like this have nothing to do with you and everything to do with the fact that *you* rising above the status quo illuminates the fact that other people are *not*.

It's much easier for people to pull you back down and commiserate with you than to rise up out of excuse-making alongside you. If fitting in and making choices that the masses understand and support is your top priority, it's going to be **very** hard to be successful at losing weight and keeping it off.

With 70% of American adults being overweight or obese, maintaining a healthy weight makes you an outlier. You likely can't look to the majority of people around you for guidance, motivation, or inspiration because they're not walking the walk. They're not on your path, but like-minded women do exist, and it's possible to find your people. Being in the minority does not mean being alone, and it helps enormously to find and surround yourself with like-minded women, as we'll talk about in Chapter 8.

Without deep *lifelong* commitment to your journey and what you want out of *your* life, it's very easy to get pulled back to the (unhealthy, unhappy) status quo.

Reminder

Being committed means deciding that your goal is important enough to stop making excuses (like most people do) and start finding solutions to whatever challenges you face. If you're tired of being in the minority, put yourself in positions where the lifestyle you want to create is already the norm.

Threat #3 To Commitment: Having a Short-Term Focus

"I've learned so much! I'm really happy with how much weight I've lost. I'm not where I want to be yet, but this was a good kickstart," Malia told me.

It was the wrap-up party for the six-week challenge that members of our gym in Hawaii had just completed in an effort to lose 10% of their body weight.

Though I was a member of the gym and was at the party to support the members I'd come to know and love, I hated pretty much everything else about these ongoing challenges.

Many participants, like Malia, were successful at losing a significant amount of weight in a short period of time. But they did so by following extremely limited meal templates that put a whole lot of "bad" foods on an off-limits pedestal and attending five rigorous workouts per week that their bodies weren't ready for, leaving them sore and desperate for rest.

Malia and I were standing next to the long, banquet-style tables that were brimming with delicious food, from malasadas to musubi, and every Hawaiian delight in between.

"What habits from the challenge will you be keeping up with now that it's over?" I asked.

"I like how it feels to come to the five a.m. class and get my workout in early. But," she continued, "my shoulder has been bothering me and I'm so sore all the time. I'm probably going to take a week off from classes."

"That makes sense," I said, "It's just as important to rest as it is to push yourself through hard workouts. What about nutrition?"

"I want to keep following the food template because it makes knowing what to eat really easy . . . but all this stuff looks sooooo good," she said, gesturing to the food. "I'll probably have a cheat day today and then get back to the template because I want to lose more weight."

Having seen several rounds of this challenge start and finish already, I knew what was in store for the majority of participants: like Malia, many would take a break from the gym—often for good reason—but very few would return. Many would struggle to continue to follow the meal template and would, instead, find themselves overeating "unapproved" foods with seemingly no self-control.

Most would end up signing up for another six-week challenge, not realizing how much it was contributing to this unhealthy (and frustrating) cycle.

If this is giving you all-or-nothing vibes, it should. Living in extremes like these challenges absolutely contributes to the starts and stops that wreck consistency.

And it's also an example of a threat to our commitment, too.

Your goal weight is not a stopping point; maintaining a healthy weight is a long-term commitment.

If you've previously approached weight loss with a willingness to do whatever it takes to see the scale drop and then want to be able to go back to your old lifestyle, beliefs, and identity, I have bad news for you: that's why your results haven't lasted.

There's no getting "there" and stopping.

Who you are now is not the person you'll be when you're maintaining a healthy weight. It's time to start seeing yourself as a fit and healthy person, rather than an overweight person desperately trying to be thin.

When you use the Gone For Good framework I'm teaching you in part 2, you won't just lose weight, you'll also become someone who has health as one of your top values—forever. You'll come to see yourself differently, as someone who already believes she *is* fit and healthy and who starts showing up in her life the way that version of herself would.

Here seems like a good place to remind you that health and weight loss are not one and the same:

You can lose weight while improving your health.

You can lose weight while worsening your health.

You can improve your health without losing weight.

You can improve your health while losing weight.

If the thought of making a long-term commitment scares you, you're not alone.

Odds are, because you've had such miserable experiences trying to lose weight in the past, you associate any sort of success with sacrifice that sounds miserable to commit to for a lifetime.

The difference after reading this book is that you'll be armed with all of the tools you need to maintain a healthy weight, while prioritizing your overall health, and enjoying your life—and the person you become—in the process.

When you aren't approaching your weight loss with an end date in mind, you give yourself the opportunity to transform how you see yourself, the world, and how you go about your day-to-day life.

The beauty is that the time you spend learning and mastering the skills and tools I'll teach you in part 2 *inherently* sets you up for long-term success. By the time you've lost the weight, it won't feel nearly as effortful to stay there.

While it won't always feel fun or easy (nothing does), anything worth having is also worth maintaining. You invest on an ongoing basis in all the other relationships you care about, and the relationship with yourself and your body is no different. Maintenance, by nature, is an ongoing process. Although this might feel daunting right now, it gets easier with time and practice, and with the healthy foundational habits you build while you're losing weight.

Part of why it feels so hard to be committed is because you don't believe that reaching your goal is possible. You've chipped away at your reputation to the point that you think you're untrustworthy, and it's hard to believe that things will be any different if you try again.

If you've found yourself in this position, you *can* repair your reputation with yourself. In the next chapter when I talk about confidence and in Chapter 9 when I teach you about compassionate ownership, you'll learn exactly how to forgive yourself for your past and become someone who does what she says she's going to do, even when no one else is looking.

Redeveloping full trust in yourself to follow through will skyrocket your commitment to your goals, as well as your overall confidence. In turn, confidence enhances consistency and commitment.

In addition, consistency helps build commitment. You won't always *feel* committed, but every time you show up for yourself and do "the things," you cast another vote for the person you want to become and further strengthen your commitment to the new version of yourself.

CHAPTER 6

CONFIDENCE

"**E**very weekend I make these big plans for the next week. I buy all these fruits and veggies so I can make green juice in the morning. I create my workout stacks on the Peloton app. I tell my husband I'm waking up early to work out before the kids . . ."

I didn't say anything when Julie paused but I knew what was coming.

"And then I don't do any of it!" she said. "Maybe I'm good for a couple days, but then a kid gets sick or I tweak my back and it all falls apart. I'm just such an all-or-nothing person, and when my plans get derailed, it takes me forever to get back on track."

After falling way short of her goals, she'd feel awful about it, then set the same goals the following week.

Julie's frustrations were understandable. It *is* hard to be consistent and committed when life is unpredictable and you're feeling pulled in a million directions.

Threat #1 To Confidence: The Impact of Not Following Through On Past Goals

If this had only happened occasionally, it wouldn't have been a big deal. But week after week, Julie would experience some version of this. Over time, she had put herself in a position where it didn't even really matter what goals she set because deep down she lacked the confidence to think she could achieve them, anyway.

She didn't realize it, but she was chipping away at her reputation with herself every time she hit snooze, bailed on a workout, went for the catered lunch instead of the one she packed, or watched one more Netflix episode even though it was bedtime.

Each of these seemingly inconsequential choices was proving to Julie that she couldn't trust herself to do what she said she'd do.

Think about how that lack of reliability would go over with your spouse, kids, or friends:

Imagine telling a friend you'd pick her up at the airport and then just deciding not to?

Imagine deciding not to get the kids from the bus because you're tired?

Imagine assuring your husband you'd pick up the dry cleaning only to instead scroll TikTok?

You wouldn't do those things because you know how important it is to be reliable and dependable. Commitments to yourself need to be treated the same way. You must be someone who does what she says she'll do, even if no one else is involved or looking.

If you've ever been in a relationship with someone who betrayed your trust, you know how difficult it is to overcome.

You have to be willing to forgive the past. You have to put yourself in positions where that person has the opportunity to prove to you that they've changed. And you have to be patient as you give yourself the time you need to really believe in your relationship again.

The same applies to your relationship with yourself. It's impossible to be confident that you'll reach a goal when you're not in the habit of showing up for yourself. Once you *start* putting yourself in the position to develop consistency and commitment, you can rebuild your self-reputation and develop confidence.

Taking action slightly outside your comfort zone is one of the best ways to build belief in yourself.

For Julie, that meant learning to be comfortable with doing *less*, at first. We scaled way back:

"What is one small goal you can set today that you're ninety-plus percent confident you can achieve? I don't care how small it is, I just want you to feel like it's a total no-brainer for you to do," I told her.

After discussing a few options, Julie settled on taking a 15-minute walk in the morning before getting ready for work. Initially resistant because she felt like running would burn more calories and, therefore, be more worthwhile, Julie realized that the thought of having to do something strenuous first thing in the morning would make her that much more likely to hit snooze. She knew from experience that waking up and moving felt good, and this felt like an easy way to start the day off on the right foot without risking setting the bar too high and falling short.

The point wasn't to make a monumental change, it was to help Julie get a win under her belt. To give her an opportunity to follow through on what she told herself she'd do, and to prove to herself that she was capable.

From there, I knew it would be that much easier for her to follow through on the next goal, and the next, even if the goals we set were getting more substantial.

Exercise, in general, is a great opportunity to get outside your comfort zone and develop confidence. Getting in the habit of working out isn't just great for your physical health; it's also one of the best ways to show yourself that you:

- can show up for yourself when you don't feel like it or it would be easier not to
- can complete a workout where none of the moves are in your wheelhouse
- can push through and give more when your brain is telling you that you can't
- are stronger than you realize

Confidence is believing that you **can**—despite the gremlins in your brain telling you otherwise.

Those experiences, that belief in yourself, transcend the walls of the gym (or guest bedroom, as the case may be) and spill over into all other areas of your life.

All that to say, if you know you're struggling with confidence, starting with exercise is a great first step toward developing it. If getting started or staying consistent has always been a challenge for you, start with less. Like Julie, set small goals you *know* you can do and won't talk yourself out of in the moment, and celebrate each time you follow through and do what you said you'd do.

If you're already exercising consistently, you may not have thought to apply that "yes I can" attitude outside of your workouts or realized the improvements it's having on your confidence. Now that it's on your radar, take notice of when you get outside your comfort zone with exercise and use that as evidence that you can learn, grow, and do hard things in other areas of your life.

Tip

If you're in the habit of falling short of your goals, set yourself up for success by setting smaller ones. Look at your consistency over the last few weeks and set the bar slightly higher than it has been, somewhere you're nine out of ten confident you can achieve even during your worst week.

Threat #2 To Confidence: Having Unrealistic Standards And Expectations

"When my plans get derailed, it takes me forever to get back on track."

That's what Julie told me in that first conversation.

What she didn't realize, at the time, was that this exact reaction to being less than perfect (aka human) was a big part of what was keeping her trapped in the all-or-nothing cycle.

She was naively expecting that as long as she knew what to eat or do for workouts, the rest would be easy. Instead of anticipating and rolling with life's inevitable curve balls, being flexible, and doing the best she could on any given day, she took these setbacks to mean that something had gone seriously wrong with her plan.

What she needed to realize was that the route to lasting weight loss is more like hiking on a mountain trail than running laps on a track.

You're not either on or off; the path just winds and is unpredictable. Sometimes it feels like a walk in the park, and sometimes you're going up a huge incline. Sometimes you'll feel like you're on the wrong trail entirely. Or like you're stuck or going in the wrong direction. Or like you've been working hard for a really long time and haven't made nearly as much progress as you were expecting.

This is all normal!

This is what the process is like for 100% of people. You just have to be willing to go where the road takes you, while staying committed to your goal and consistent in the actions it'll take to get you there.

There's nothing wrong with you if you've experienced being "off track." Don't make the ups and downs mean anything about you or your ability to be successful. They're *actually* opportunities to learn new skills, build resilience, and be better equipped to handle the next setback more easily and with less disruption.

Using these experiences as evidence that there's something wrong with you and you'll never be able to reach and maintain a healthy weight is only exacerbating your lack of confidence, which ultimately becomes a self-fulfilling prophecy.

To quote Henry Ford, "Whether you believe you can do a thing or not, you are right."

You don't have to know what to do 100% of the time, but you do need to believe in yourself enough to try and trust that you can figure it out. Only by putting yourself on the hiking trail and putting one foot in front of the other are you able to develop confidence and reach your goals.

There will be times when all you want to do is whine and complain about how unfair things are. That's okay. You're allowed to feel and express those emotions.

Once you have, and it's time to show up regardless of how you're feeling, all you have to do is "parent yourself" into doing the damn thing. Just like you'd tell an actual toddler, "Too bad, this is what we're doing," sometimes you need to give yourself the same tough love.

Threat #3 To Confidence: Past Negative Experiences

My client, Jackie, grew up with a mom who was obsessed with how she looked, seldom eating anything besides cottage cheese and often leaving the kids for hours on end to go to Jazzercise. From a young age, she picked up on the message that being thin is of the utmost importance, so the extra weight she was carrying around since having kids really did a number on her confidence.

Now a mom herself, she was very cautious about never putting her own needs before those of her family, as she felt her mom had done too often. As a result, she had a tendency to just go with the flow when it came to restaurant choices or how to spend their free time, never wanting to rock the boat by suggesting something that would help her prioritize her health goals but could be perceived as selfish.

Another client, Casey, grew up in an active family, playing multiple sports and taking vacations full of hiking and zip lining. Although weight gain in adulthood left her not looking or performing like the athlete she once was, she still identified as an athlete and worked out consistently because the habit was so well established by then.

On the other hand, my client Emmie's early experiences with exercise felt traumatic. Memories of middle school were riddled with the sting of being picked last in gym class, being targeted during dodgeball, and being the last to finish the one-mile run during the Presidential Physical Fitness Challenge. These experiences took a toll on her confidence and resulted in a rocky relationship with exercise as an adult that she had to work to improve during our time together.

These are just a few of many examples of the life experiences that are having an impact on your confidence today and the success—or lack thereof—you've experienced with weight loss so far.

How you've ended up here is a product of your entire life leading up to this point. All your past experiences, positive and negative, play a role in how you feel about yourself, how you perceive other people, and how you view the world.

Everything from the comment your grandfather made about you being "solid" when he picked you up as a kid (just me?), to the things your mom would say about herself and her body when she didn't know you were listening (or worse, when she did), have helped shape the person you are today.

Everything from the positive attention you got when you lost weight to the deep, dark reasons you used food to hide in your own body, has helped shape the person you are today.

Everything from whether your first experience working out at a gym was positive or negative, and whether your spouse and friends are encouraging and supportive or disparaging and discouraging has shaped the person you are today.

I know and understand that it can take time to identify, untangle, and unlearn these messages and beliefs. It's something I'll help you do in Chapter 9 when we talk about compassionate ownership.

Whether or not you believe it right now, I want you to know that you are not your weight. You are worthy and deserving of love, success, and all the things, regardless of the number on the scale.

If you think losing weight is the key to worthiness, love, affection, success, or happiness, you're going to be in for a rude awakening when you reach your weight-loss goal only to find that none of that other stuff has changed.

Let me be clear: you can be confident at any size. Losing weight is not going to inherently improve your confidence. There's not a number on the scale under which you magically turn on your confidence. The confidence you gain when you lose weight with the Gone For Good formula is because of the person you become in the process and the work you do to disentangle this mental mess.

You cannot hate yourself into a smaller size, and trying to will *not* improve your confidence, regardless of how much weight you lose.

The key to building confidence while losing weight is that lasting change has to start from within, from a place of love and acceptance, which this book will help you do.

As adults and as moms or role models for our own kids or other important children in our lives, we have such an opportunity to give our own children many gifts we may not have received as children.

We have the opportunity to set a better example than was set for us.

To learn how to speak about our bodies the way we'd like the next generation of girls to speak about their own.

To instill the belief that exercise and movement are luxuries that we *get* to do, not *have* to do in order to look a certain way.

To understand that it's okay to use food for comfort and celebration—and *also* have a full skill set of other tools and coping mechanisms to use when those would be better for us.

To normalize eating fruits, veggies, and lean proteins because they're filled with important nutrients that our bodies need in order to be strong, healthy, and happy—and *also* to know it's okay to indulge in foods that just taste good.

To remember it's not about eating as little as possible but learning how to fuel our bodies for our lifestyles and understand all the benefits of a healthy life that have nothing to do with size.

If this sounds idealistic and daunting, like it would be hard to teach children these things because you don't even know how to do them yourself, you're not alone. You don't have to feel confident in doing all these things in order to start, and once you *do* start, your confidence will grow.

As adults, we're not in the habit of putting ourselves in positions where we need to learn new things. It can be scary and uncomfortable.

You'll want to skip that part, but you can't. You need to be willing to be a beginner.

Staying consistent in the beginning—and staying committed when the going gets tough—is what creates the confidence that separates the successful few from the masses.

A few things can help immensely with this: setting smaller goals, having support to work through challenges while noticing and celebrating your wins, and having the external accountability to help stay focused when you're vulnerable to giving up.

For Julie, and all my clients in the beginning of coaching, having someone to check in with who will help them navigate life, make sure they're following through, and help them see the things that are going well makes all the difference in the world when it comes to staying consistent, committed, and developing the confidence to believe that reaching their goals is inevitable. The combination of these will help you to get early wins under your belt, build the momentum to tackle additional changes, and get to a place where you're powered by habit and intrinsic motivation.

Tip

In addition to the suggestions above, you may benefit from additional mental health support to work through childhood trauma as it relates to your confidence and feelings of worthiness.

There won't be an exact moment where you arrive at Confidence; it'll happen gradually over time, and you'll notice that you don't doubt yourself as much and that it's just easier to follow through on decisions that help you shift your identity to that of a fit and healthy person.

Confidence comes from being faced with challenges, from doing your best to overcome them even though you know that means you might "fail" or mess up, from reflecting back with compassion for yourself, from seeing what lessons you can learn, and from trying again.

Confidence won't make it effortless to maintain your weight, but having developed skills, tools, resilience, grit, and strength along the way will position you with everything you need to overcome whatever obstacle stands in your way, both now and in the future.

The following journaling prompts will help you try on the identity of someone who is more confident by considering the possibility that reaching your goals *is* possible for you. They're a way to become aware of the negative stories you may be telling yourself and to test out alternative thoughts that will help you show up as the most confident version of yourself.

Journal Prompts

This exercise is great for getting to the root of why you're doubting your ability to lose weight permanently, and to start trying on the identity of someone who already has.

Set a timer for 10 minutes.

Goal: _____

Confidence at achieving that goal (on a scale of 1-10): ____

Commitment to achieving that goal (on a scale of 1-10): ___

(It is fine, and expected, if you're nowhere near a 10 for either of these).

Write down all the reasons you're feeling like a _____ (number).

This will be a list of all your self-doubts (i.e., "I don't think I can. I'll probably give up. I don't know how.")

_____

_____

_____

_____

_____

_____

_____

Once you've emptied your brain of those, ask yourself, "If I was ten out of ten confident that I would achieve this goal, or I already had, what thoughts would I be having then?"

This allows you to entertain the idea of being able to do the thing. (i.e., "I know what to do. I work hard. I have everything I need. I give my best. I've done lots of hard things.")

_____

_____

_____

_____

_____

_____

_____

Do this EVERY DAY for 30 days, and I guarantee it will change so much of how you're thinking about yourself and the results you're getting in return.

Breaking Up with The Parts of
Your Old Self That Are No Longer Serving You

It's likely that these parts of you are what's holding you back from reaching your weight-loss goals and your true potential.

Your Old Self is trying to help you, but she's misguided. She thinks that she's helping you by protecting you from failure, but she's really keeping you stuck.

She's the one who doubts you at every turn. Who allows you to keep putting everyone and everything before yourself. Who keeps self-sabotaging and makes you feel like you can't get out of your own way.

Your Old Self may have served you in the past, but it's time to take what you need from her and make room for a new version of yourself: Your BEST Self.

It's time to write a breakup letter to the parts of your Old Self that are no longer serving you. It's time to move forward and become the best version of yourself.

Here is a visualization to help you identify, sort, and declutter your mind:

Close your eyes and visualize your brain as an attic cluttered with a lifetime's worth of stuff.

It's full of junk. Mostly crap you don't need but haven't gotten around to throwing away. Lyrics to songs that you haven't heard in 15 years. That embarrassing thing that happened in high school. The comeback you didn't think of until it was too late. The hair and fashion styles that you wish went undocumented. You get the idea. There's just a lot of crap taking up space up there.

Including the boxes of "Things That Are Holding Me Back," full of aaaall the stuff preventing you from moving forward on your weight loss and lifestyle transformation journey.

Things That Are Holding You Back:

- The mean girls in middle school calling you "fat"
- Being picked last in gym
- Your mom putting you on a diet at a young age
- Being really fit pre-kids, something you think you'll never achieve again
- Clothes that you think you'll never fit into again
- Negative self-talk about why you can't achieve your goals

What ridiculous clutter do you still have taking up mental space in your brain that you can get rid of today? Are those memories or experiences really worth saving, holding onto, or continuing to dwell on?

NO! They're not serving you!

Write out that letter to your Old Self and get rid of that mental clutter that's been holding you back for way too long.

_____

_____

_____

_____

_____

_____

_____

Postcard From Your Future Self

It's time to look toward the future.

To stop defining yourself by what you're scared of or want to avoid and to start becoming your Best Self.

In order to figure out what the best version of You is like, make a list of what you want.

Here are some examples:

I want to be lean, healthy, and muscular.

I want to be strong, fast, flexible, and physically capable of doing the things I enjoy.

I want to take fewer medications, or get off my medications entirely.

I want to feel comfortable and confident in the gym.

I want to try new activities and have new experiences.

I want to be healthy, mobile, and pain-free. I want to feel like I'm thriving.

I want to feel sexy.

I want to not obsess about food. I want to nourish my body with good food choices most of the time and not beat myself up when I choose to indulge.

_____

_____

_____

_____

_____

_____

_____

If you're struggling with figuring out what you want, try starting with a list of what you don't want:

I don't want to feel out of shape.

I don't want to take all these medications.

I don't want to feel uncomfortable in the gym.

I don't want to be achy and sore all the time.

I don't want to feel out of control of my eating.

_____

_____

_____

_____

_____

_____

If you don't want to feel out of control with your eating, then you do want to make food choices that are aligned with your goals and make you feel good.

Once you know what you want in the future, imagine you get a postcard.

It's from your Future Self, and it's showing you what your future looks like. This book is the beginning of the journey to becoming that version of yourself.

One year from today, in an ideal world, what is your Future Self doing?

Where is your Future Self (physically, with her job, in relationships, etc.)?

What is your Future Self doing (literally, how does she spend her days/weeks)?

How does your Future Self feel (about herself, her life, her loved ones, her job, etc.)?

How does your Future Self respond to "life" getting in the way of what she wants (e.g. inconveniences, illnesses, long work hours, fighting kids, bad weather, etc.)?

What behaviors does your Future Self engage in on a regular basis?

What adventures is your Future Self having?

Forget being realistic. Just imagine who and where you could be one year from now if you were your Future Self.

Sit down and write out that postcard from your Future Self.

_____

_____

_____

_____

_____

_____

_____

_____

With that, you've completed Part 1—the 3 Cs of Success!

So far we've covered the four main reasons why it's so hard to lose weight and keep it off for good:

1. Diets encourage restriction, deprivation, and an all-or-nothing mentality.
2. Most weight-loss programs are impersonal, isolating, and rely on negativity to fuel surface-level change.
3. The modern world is tailored to make it hard to maintain a healthy weight.
4. Blame culture makes it easy to shirk responsibility.

We've explored the top threats to consistency, commitment, and confidence—the 3 Cs of success:

- Threat #1 To Health Consistency: All-Or-Nothing Approach
- Threat #2 To Health Consistency: Flying Under The Radar
- Threat #3 To Health Consistency: Expectation Management

- Threat #1 To Commitment: Vague And Surface-Level Goals
- Threat #2 to Commitment: Being In The Minority
- Threat #3 To Commitment: Having A Short-Term Focus

- Threat #1 To Confidence: The Impact Of Not Following Through On Past Goals

- Threat #2 To Confidence: Having Unrealistic Standards And Expectations
- Threat #3 To Confidence: Past Negative Experiences

Now it's time to dive into my Gone For Good formula that will help you learn and master the exercise and nutrition "Big Rocks," see the value of having comprehensive support, and learn how to take compassionate ownership of your weight-loss journey. In turn, these will help you develop the consistency, commitment, and confidence you need to reach your weight-loss goal, for good.

PART 2

INTRODUCING THE GONE
FOR GOOD FRAMEWORK

The next few chapters will simplify exactly *what* to do to develop consistency, commitment, and confidence in pursuit of your goal to lose weight and keep it off, *while* prioritizing your overall health, happiness, and well-being.

Although everyone's circumstances are unique, most women experience similar roadblocks that get in the way of the 3 Cs of success for lasting weight loss:

- Falling into the all-or-nothing trap
- Second-guessing whether you're doing it "right"
- Not having anyone to hold you accountable so you fall off after a couple weeks and not knowing where to turn for advice and guidance when you're struggling
- Not having people around you who support you and want to grow with you
- Being easily derailed by "life stuff"
- Feeling like a victim or like what you do won't matter anyway

The list above, and whatever else you would add, can be categorized into and addressed with three distinct areas of focus that will help you become more consistent, committed, and confident—the three pillars of my Gone For Good formula: learning and mastering the exercise and nutrition "Big Rocks," having comprehensive support, and taking compassionate ownership of the process.

86 To Your Health

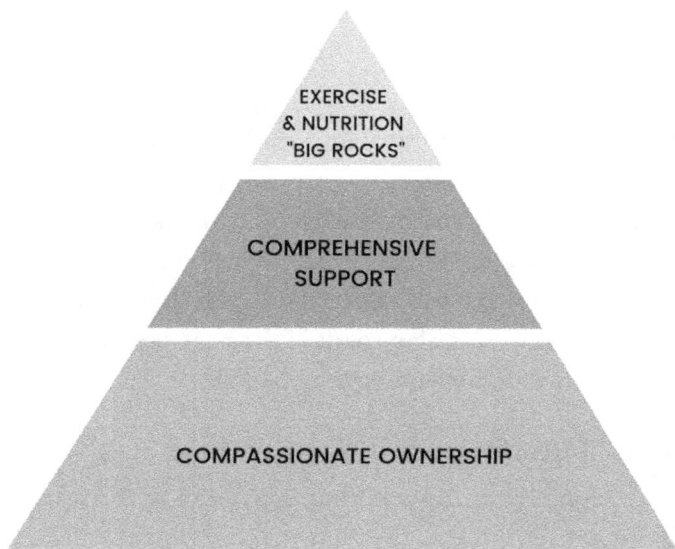

Pillar 1: Learning & Mastering the "Big Rocks"

Pareto Principle

For many outcomes, roughly 80% of consequences come from 20% of causes.

Most women approach weight loss by either trying to focus on everything at once, including things that are inconsequential, or things I consider "pebbles," like whether they should fast and for how long, how many meals to eat, or which Peloton rides are best for weight loss. Or focusing on *just* those "pebbles," which leaves them feeling overwhelmed and frustrated by their lack of results.

For lasting weight loss, the majority of results come from focusing on the most effective forms of movement and top nutrition priorities to maximize your results, a handful of key behaviors that I call the "Big Rocks": **daily movement, strength training, rest & recovery, calories, protein, and fiber.**

Learning and mastering them allows you to simplify, focus on doing less, and address whatever obstacles stand in the way of doing them consistently. The result is that you'll get better results that feel more sustainable, with less effort.

To help you understand the relationship between the "Big Rocks" and the "pebbles," remember the jar analogy from Chapter 1. If you fill your jar with small things like "pebbles" and sand, it'll take a really long time and a lot of energy to fill it up (if you don't give up in frustration first)!

Filling your jar first with the "Big Rocks" we're covering next allows you to do so efficiently by prioritizing the most impactful behaviors that generate the majority of your results. After that—and only if you *want*—you can focus on the smaller "pebbles."

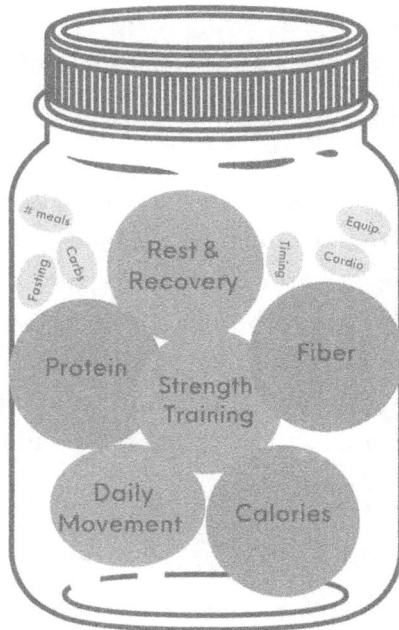

In Chapters 7 and 8 we'll dive into why the three exercise "Big Rocks" and three nutrition "Big Rocks" are so important and how to implement them in your life until you've mastered them and they feel routine.

Actually implementing these six habits into your lifestyle needn't be a sequential thing, and you can tackle them in whatever order makes sense for you. Although nutrition choices are really what drive weight loss (or lack thereof), I've decided to address exercise first because it's simpler to outline and easy to implement right away. This can help you get some wins under your belt, build momentum, and feel more confident tackling your nutrition, which may feel like more of an undertaking.

Pillar 2: Comprehensive Support

> *"You are the average of the five people*
> *you spend the most time with."*
> —*Jim Rohn*

Turns out, it's not just your close friends who influence you; a study[5] found that friends of friends of friends can have influence on whether or not we smoke, how much we weigh, and how happy we are. Whether you've realized it or not, the people around you are having a big impact on your lifestyle.

As such, it's incredibly important to be intentional about with whom you surround yourself. It'll be much easier to be

---

[5] https://www.nejm.org/doi/full/10.1056/NEJMsa066082

in the minority of women who lose weight and keep it off when you choose to be around people who can help guide you, support you, inspire you, and help normalize the lifestyle changes you want to make.

I know it can be hard to make deliberate choices about who to spend your time with, and even harder to reach out for professional help once you realize you'd benefit from more guidance and accountability than your peers can offer.

I can relate; when I first started my business, I spent *years* stubbornly trying to do it all alone. I had the mentality that needing help was a sign of weakness or admitting defeat and that I should be able to figure it out on my own.

Many of my clients feel similarly before eventually reaching out to me for support in their weight-loss journey. We're used to shouldering all sorts of burdens and responsibilities while pretending they're no big deal; meanwhile, we're silently drowning.

Now that I've come to believe that asking for help is a sign of strength, I'm quick to seek out the support that I need. On a sales call for a book-writing mentorship, I was asked what I felt was holding me back from reaching my goals. I was pleasantly surprised by my response: "I know I can do it, but I also know it would be faster and easier to follow the path of someone who's done it before and to have a community of support along the way."

That program is the same one that helped me get this book into your hands, and the guidance, support, and accountability *was* invaluable. I was able to avoid the rookie pitfalls most novice authors run into, I had unwavering support from other women walking the same path, my inevitable challenges were met with understanding and helpful advice, and I got to share my wins with dozens of women who celebrated them as their own. The whole process was smoother and more enjoyable than if I'd tried to do it alone.

In Chapter 9, we'll dive into who you need in your corner to reach your goals, where to find them, and how to reconsider and recalibrate relationships along the way.

Pillar 3: Compassionate Ownership

Compassionate Ownership

Being empathetic toward yourself and your circumstances while also recognizing and taking responsibility for the things in your life you can control: your thoughts, attitude, and behaviors.

Most women aren't thinking about how to maintain their results when they embark on a weight-loss journey. And as a result, they find it very hard to do so.

When you tackle excess weight with the Gone For Good formula, you develop the self-awareness to get to the root of why you're struggling and cultivate the growth mindset to develop the skills and tools that will help you overcome those challenges—and any in the future—that stand in your way. This may mean learning how to set better boundaries, develop better time-management skills, or improve your self-talk so you're no longer your own worst enemy.

It's absolutely essential to develop the skill of compassionate ownership; this is where you cement your results for life.

We'll cover compassionate ownership in depth in Chapter 10.

I'm excited for you to learn my formula because I know it'll make reaching your goals and staying there so much more attainable. Let's get started!

CHAPTER 7

EXERCISE "BIG ROCKS"

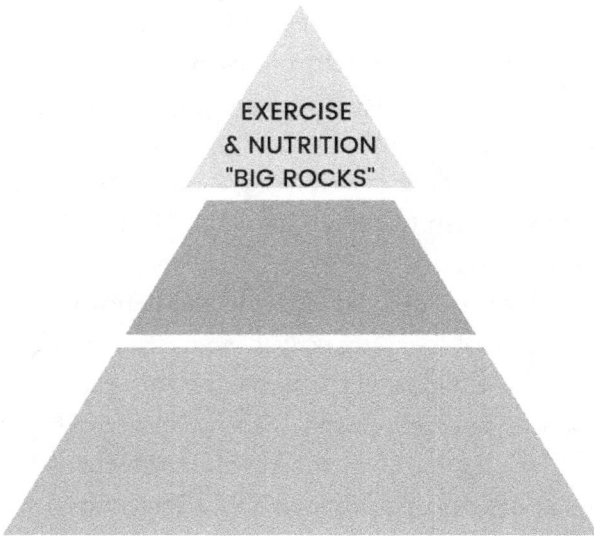

Tanya and I met *after* she'd already lost a considerable amount of weight on her own. She was incredibly proud of her accomplishment, not the least of which was being more consistent with working out than she'd ever been in her life.

Every morning since January, she resisted the temptation to hit snooze and stay warm and cozy for just a few more minutes. She was up at the crack of dawn to start her nearly two-hour daily cardio routine she was using to try to offset being sedentary the entire rest of the day.

Initially, it felt great. She was proud of her commitment to get up when it would have been so much easier not to. She could feel the previous day's stressors melting away as the calorie count on her treadmill ticked up. Seeing the scale drop each week only motivated her to workout harder and longer.

One of the things she was most proud of was her activity "streak" and the fact that it meant she hadn't missed a day of working out for the better part of a year.

Tanya reached out to me in August, and although she was maintaining her initial weight loss, she felt weak, tired, irritable, and incredibly frustrated that she had stalled out and stopped losing, despite remaining incredibly consistent with her workouts.

She felt like she needed the calorie burn for stress relief, but now much of her stress was *about* her workouts. She was constantly anxious that she would somehow miss a day and break her coveted streak. She was incredibly hard on herself if she wasn't able to hit a Personal Record (PR) each workout, or at least push herself harder than she had the previous day, but that was getting harder and harder to do. It was like her body just couldn't do what it could just a few months prior.

She had nagging aches and pains that she'd been ignoring for months but feared would turn into some sort of major injury that would put her right back on the couch.

Tanya's experience is an example of the all too common all-or-nothing mentality we've talked about earlier. While her behaviors didn't feel extreme at first, she'd been "all in" for a long time, and it was taking an obvious toll. Fortunately, Tanya's experience is completely avoidable.

I knew Tanya could get the rest of the weight off without continuing to run herself into the ground with grueling, hours-long cardio sessions. All she needed was to prioritize the exercise "Big Rocks" I'm sharing with you in this and the next chapter.

The exercise and nutrition "Big Rocks" are the tip of the three-layer pyramid for a reason.

Although they're incredibly important, and you won't lose weight without having them aligned with your goals, they're actually the simplest piece of the lasting weight-loss puzzle.

Before we talk about the specifics of the three exercise "Big Rocks": daily movement, strength training, and rest & recovery, let's go over some quick definitions to make sure we're on the same page. In order to lose weight, you must be in a caloric deficit, which is to say that your body is using more calories than it's taking in. In this chapter, we're focusing on the "calories out" side of this weight-loss equation:

Total Calories out > Total Calories in = Weight Loss

Metabolism: The chemical processes that occur within a living organism in order to maintain life.

Odds are, you've heard a lot of myths and misconceptions about your metabolism. Many of these start off with a tiny bit of truth that ends up getting blown out of proportion, sort of like a game of telephone.

One example is the myth of "starvation mode." It's true that your body wants to survive and will attempt to maintain homeostasis. As such, your metabolism is adaptive and responds to how much energy (calories) you're taking in. When you're taking in fewer calories, your metabolism will "down regulate" in an effort to match the energy going out with the energy coming in. This dynamic is part of why losing weight, in practice, isn't as straightforward as the equation above may make it seem.

To be clear: this downregulation is normal, you won't experience it to a huge degree, you can't "break" your metabolism, and eating too little will never cause you to gain weight or be unable to lose it (prisoners of war, among others, prove that eating way too little over an extended period of time will, in fact, lead to actual starvation).

When you refer to your metabolism, you're likely talking about your **basal metabolic rate (BMR),** or the calories you burn just to survive while basically being in a vegetative state (like keeping your organs functioning), which make up 70% of the total calories you burn each day. (Let's call these "staying alive" calories).

There are actually 3 more components to your **total daily energy expenditure (TDEE),** which is the sum of all the energy (calories) you use. This is the amount of energy (calories) that will help you maintain your current weight:

Thermic Effect of Food (TEF)—calories burned digesting food you eat, 10% (digestive calories)

Exercise activity thermogenesis (EAT)—calories you burn during intentional exercise, 5% (workout calories)

Non-exercise activity thermogenesis (NEAT)—calories you burn through daily movement outside of exercise, 15% (daily movement calories)

**COMPONENTS OF TOTAL DAILY
ENERGY EXPENDITURE (TDEE)**

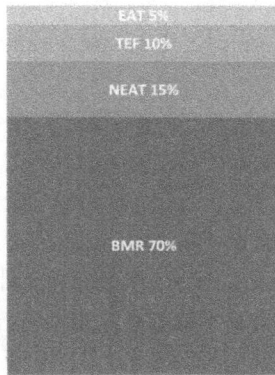

EAT 5%

TEF 10%

NEAT 15%

BMR 70%

You may be surprised to see that exercise is such a small piece of your total energy expenditure! This largely boils down to the fact that no matter how intensely you're exercising, you're still doing it for a short period of time. The calories you burn during your workouts are often offset by being less active outside of them or by taking in more calories the rest of the day.

I hope it's a relief to see that your *non*-exercise movement (NEAT) has a larger impact on your daily calorie needs. Just taking up active hobbies, playing with your kids or pets, doing chores and running errands are contributing to the calories you burn and can help you lose weight!

As you can see, your BMR is the largest contributor to your total daily energy (calorie) needs, at 70%, but it's also the component you have the least control over.

Aside from building muscle (which is a little more energetically expensive than other tissues), the only way to increase your BMR is to have a bigger body—aka the opposite of losing weight.

In fact, as you lose weight and your body becomes smaller, your BMR also decreases and the caloric intake that was previously eliciting weight loss becomes your maintenance intake.

You needn't focus much on TEF (let's call them digestive calories so it's a little easier to remember), as it's a pretty small piece of the puzzle. Just know that some foods (proteins) require more energy to digest and absorb than others, so prioritizing those foods can make a small difference in your calorie burn throughout the day. Another consideration that complicates the weight-loss equation is that being in a caloric deficit (aka taking in less food, as is necessary to lose weight) means needing less energy to digest and absorb it. As you reduce calories, you expend even less energy digesting those calories, and so on.

How many calories you're burning during your workouts (we'll call them workout calories) is where most women focus their attention when it comes to daily movement. Like digestive calories, this is also a pretty small piece of the weight loss puzzle.

The most variable component of your total daily energy expenditure is NEAT, which, like I mentioned earlier, is all the stuff you do throughout the day *outside* of your workouts, like walking around, taking the stairs, playing with your kids, doing chores, and more (we'll call this daily movement calories).

Thanks to modern conveniences like grocery delivery, high speed internet so we can work from home in our jammies, and non-stop streaming services like Netflix, we have to be a lot more intentional about our daily movement than in previous generations.

Like many women at the beginning of the coronavirus pandemic, you may have been frustrated that you were exercising *more* (thanks to not having a commute and in-home equipment like Peloton), but you still weren't losing weight (or were maybe even gaining).

Where previously you were walking to and from your car or train, running errands, heading down the hall for a meeting with coworkers, pacing up and down the field at your kid's sporting events, suddenly you were doing none of that.

While you may have slightly increased the calories you were burning through exercise, it was offset by the fact that your daily movement plummeted.

With that context, here are the exercise "Big Rocks" for women looking to lose fat while improving overall health and fitness:

1. Daily movement (often in the form of a step goal)
2. Strength training
3. Rest & recovery

You might be surprised that cardiovascular exercise isn't on this list. Rather than a Big Rock, cardio is more of a Pebble: it can be great for your health and has a ton of benefits. If you enjoy it, keep doing it.

That said, most women I've encountered in the last 20 years over-focus on cardio (especially the high-intensity variety) to the detriment of other forms of movement—like the "Big Rocks"—that would actually benefit them more and help them reach their weight-loss goals more successfully. Let's go over each one in more detail.

Exercise Big Rock #1: Daily Movement

Part of what Tanya was missing was a focus on developing a more active lifestyle *outside* of her workouts. Though her morning calorie burn might have been admirable, it was offset by the fact that she was sitting or sleeping the entire rest of the day. Her exercise (EAT) calories had increased, but her daily movement (NEAT) calories remained quite low, even lower, in fact, than they'd been before her morning workouts because now she was too tired to play with her dog or garden after work.

Assuming you're able to walk safely and comfortably, a daily step goal puts an emphasis on general movement and helps increase your daily activity. Not just that, but walking also has dozens of other important benefits for anyone wanting to be generally healthy: reduction in anger and hostility, improved cardiovascular health, reduced risk of chronic diseases, less joint pain, better decision-making, stronger bones, and better immune and digestive systems, to name a few.

If you're unable to walk for any reason, there are still ways to increase your daily movement, even if you're still seated, for example, the woman in my Facebook group who uses a wheelchair and goes out for "wheels" most days.

Without intention, most of us may only take a few thousand steps or have a handful of active moments per day, especially if you work from home and enjoy sedentary hobbies. Our lives are set up to be inactive and we need to be active participants in making sure that's not the case.

So how many steps should you be taking or how much should you be moving?

There's no specific threshold for how active you need to be to lose weight or be healthy. In fact, regardless of how you choose to move your body outside your workouts, the important thing to remember is to meet yourself where you are and gradually increase daily movement from there.

As an example, the common target of 10,000 daily steps does give you something relatively difficult to strive for, but there's no magic that happens at 10,000 as opposed to 9,999.

And actually, that benchmark originated as part of a marketing campaign for a Japanese pedometer because the character for 10,000 looks kind of like a person walking:

10,000   万

When it comes to setting *your* goal, I've found, personally, and with clients, that consistently getting over 8,000 steps is usually a pretty good indicator that you're making an effort to move more than you would otherwise. This would be the equivalent of about 90 minutes of movement, often broken up into small chunks of a few minutes here and there throughout the day.

There's really no upper limit to how much walking or movement you can or should do, so I would focus on starting where you are and increase gradually until 8,000 daily steps or about 90 minutes of moving around throughout the day is your minimum, understanding that your movement will fluctuate day to day.

What to do: Use your smartphone, watch, or a digital pedometer and start tracking your daily steps or active time.

Look at your average across a whole week, as well as for any outlier days that are much higher or lower than your norm.

Set a daily step or movement goal that is 500-1,000 steps or 5-10 minutes above your previous week's average and strive for that for as long as it takes to make it your new normal.

Continue increasing by small amounts until you're consistently around the benchmarks above.

(Beware of the all-or-nothing mentality creeping in. Remember to treat these recommendations as guidelines, not benchmarks that are set in stone. The day is not a failure if you "only" walk 7,000 steps; the goal is just to lead a consistently active lifestyle, so do your best to move as much as is feasible and don't major in the minors.)

Exercise Big Rock #2: Strength Training

Tanya was unfamiliar with weights, so she shied away from them. Occasionally she'd pick up a pair of light dumbbells and do some arm work, but otherwise she stuck to what she knew: her spin bike and treadmill.

She hated how her muffin top looked in her work pants; she did a lot of core work but felt like she couldn't tell the difference, anyway.

Because she didn't really know how to lift weights, it wasn't nearly as fun or engaging as the cardio she enjoyed, and she wasn't getting the results from lifting that other people seemed to rave about. It didn't really seem worth doing.

Despite many more women strength training than in previous generations, there are still a lot of misconceptions I want to address so that you feel confident and comfortable lifting in a way that supports your weight-loss and health goals.

You may have heard that muscle burns more calories than fat. This is true, but not to the extent you may be thinking. A pound of muscle burns about six calories per day, while fat only burns two to three calories. Certainly not a huge difference when it comes to a single pound of one or the other, but it does start to add up when you gradually reduce fat while building muscle (called body recomposition) over months and years.

While the "extra" calorie burn that muscle offers may be underwhelming, the extent to which prioritizing strength training can change the look of your body (not to mention your physical capabilities) is anything but.

Hypertrophy, another term for building muscle, helps you avoid reaching your goal only to find that you're "skinny fat," still having a high percentage of body fat despite having lost weight on the scale and no longer being considered overweight. Lifting also helps you look leaner, reduce loose skin after significant weight loss, and generally feel like a badass who's capable of doing life (like carrying heavy groceries) more easily. Not to mention, it's incredibly important for women to be strong and have muscle as we age and naturally start to lose it, become more prone to brittle bones, and more.

If you've been dipping your toes into the strength-training waters by going to Orangetheory, following a Pinterest routine, or adding Peloton Intervals & Arms classes into the mix, great! Picking classes or workouts at random is fine, and any strength training is better than none.

But a few tweaks to the approach most women take to strength training can skyrocket what you get out of it (which will make you actually want to keep doing it). As a bonus, I've also included a 30-day program in your online portal that includes video demos of all the exercises and a workout tracker you can print.

Focusing on major muscle groups—If you're new to lifting or if you're not sure you can commit to doing more than three days per week (which is plenty and actually my recommended goal), stick with total body sessions that target the major muscle groups, rather than worrying about a "split" program where you may be isolating small muscle groups like arms and core. If you're consistently lifting four or more days, splitting into upper body days and lower body days makes sense to allow for recovery.

Lifting heavy enough—It's time to stop picking up your 40-pound kids, only to work out using three-pound paperweights. In general, shooting for 6-12 repetitions (reps) per set is a good range for those of us lifting for overall health and weight loss.

You want to feel like you only have 1-2 reps left in the tank before your form starts to falter. If you're able to get 12 reps at a certain weight without sacrificing form, that's a sign to increase your weight on the next set or workout. When you do, get as many reps as you can and gradually work your way up again.

Starting Weights Recommendations

If you're new to lifting and unsure what weights to start with, I recommend getting three sets of dumbbells: 5, 10, and 15 pounds. This will allow you to learn proper lifting form while challenging muscle groups of different sizes and strengths. (Larger muscle groups will be able to lift heavier weights than smaller ones).

Within your first year of lifting, you'll likely be ready to increase some of your weights to 20-25 pounds or heavier.

Following a progressive program—Progressive overload is when you gradually increase the weight, reps, sets, or frequency of your lifting workouts. A progressive program will have you repeating workouts to give yourself the opportunity to continue to challenge your body even as it adapts to the stimulus so you continue seeing results.

This progression is the key to getting stronger and building muscle, so it should be considered a non-negotiable.

Exercise Big Rock #3: Rest & Recovery

Tanya's biggest issue was her fear of rest days. She was incredibly fearful of breaking her streak, and not just because she was relying on burning 1,000-plus calories every morning. Her (misguided) all-or-nothing tendencies had her convinced that one missed day would be the beginning of the end and before she knew it, months would have gone by, she'd have regained all the weight, and she'd be right back where she started.

Rest days are really important; they're when your body has a chance to recover and benefit from the hard work you're putting in during your workouts and reduce your risk of injury.

"Rest" doesn't necessarily mean doing literally nothing all day, but you should be taking days off from taxing workouts. Your brain might be happier calling them "active recovery" days, where you focus on restorative movement like yoga, stretching, and walking (you don't need rest days from your step goal), while giving your body a break from intense strength training or cardio.

Rest days can also be great opportunities to set yourself up for nutritional success by taking the time you *would* have spent exercising and using it to meal plan or prep, grocery shop, or clean up your kitchen.

Without knowing what *your* workouts look like and how well your overall lifestyle supports recovering from them, I can't prescribe exactly how many rest days are optimal for you each week, but the answer is at least one (and likely more). Learning when to push and when to rest comes with practice, but when you follow the exercise guidelines in this chapter, you'll experience the benefits of being more intentional and doing less, recovering more fully, and seeing better results.

Your workouts aren't the only consideration when it comes to determining the optimal number of rest days. Your nutrition (whether you're eating enough to support your activity level), hydration, sleep, and stress management all play a role. Since most of us have relatively high stress levels, forget to drink enough water, neglect sleep, and intentionally eat less than our body would like in order to lose weight, odds are you're not recovering well.

When you start building in rest, even preemptively when you don't feel like you need it, your body will thank you, you'll see better results, and you'll be less likely to end up burned out or injured.

Every single healthy person I know who's been consistently active for years on end takes rest days (usually because they've learned the hard way), and resting is *not* a sign of laziness or lack of commitment—quite the opposite! Tanya eventually came around to this realization, as well, after using an upcoming cruise as an opportunity to take a few days off. After coming home feeling rejuvenated and hitting a Personal Record (PR) on her Peloton, she started incorporating active rest days and "deload" (shorter, less intense) weeks into her workout routine.

Exercise "Big Rocks" Overview

Working out and being active is incredibly important for overall health and doesn't need to be confusing or time consuming. Keeping it simple and focusing on these "Big Rocks" allows you to develop habits and routines that make movement a constant in your life while freeing up more mental energy to focus on your nutrition and other lifestyle factors that have a larger impact on your goals (like nutrition, which we'll cover in the next chapter).

I recommend working your way up to a simple exercise framework where you:

1. Big Rock #1: Walk at least 8,000 steps per day (or whatever equivalent of daily movement works for you).

2. Big Rock #2: Prioritize strength two to four times per week.

3. Big Rock #3: Build in a yoga class, stretch, or rest day or two.

4. Pebbles: If you have the time and desire, feel free to add in one to four cardio sessions per week of varying modalities, lengths, and intensities—as you enjoy. (If there are other forms of movement you enjoy, adjust the frequency or duration of your "Big Rocks" to allow yourself time to incorporate them in without neglecting rest).

Action Items

Get (or start using) an activity tracker to track your daily movement/steps. Work on gradually increasing over the next few months.

Write down and commit to your new workout schedule based on the framework above.

Lifestyle Factors

Veronica felt like she was working 24/7. Her job monopolized all of her time. Because she's also a single mom, that meant starting super early in the morning so she had time to get her three kids to school, holding meetings in the car or on the sidelines of the soccer field, and completing late night reports after the kids went to bed. Feeling pulled in so many directions meant her own self-care was far on the back burner—and had been for more than a decade.

She was in the habit of drinking her first two cups of coffee while checking email before the sun came up, skipping breakfast in the mad dash to get everyone out the door on time, living on more coffee and the occasional energy drink to get her through the workday, and rarely eating anything before picking the kids up from school. After she got the kids to bed at night, she'd find herself in the pantry eating cookies and sugary treats that gave her a boost of energy and felt like the only opportunity she had all day to do something for herself. She'd work late into the night with a glass (or three) of wine in bed until she finally went to sleep around two a.m., only to start the whole routine over in just a handful of hours.

She signed up for coaching with me after a panic attack landed her in the hospital and made her realize that her current lifestyle was not just unsustainable, but downright dangerous.

She knew she couldn't keep burning the candle at both ends and ignoring all her body's signals that she was running herself into the ground. But at the same time, she didn't know what or how to change. She felt stuck.

I knew before we tackled the exercise and nutrition "Big Rocks," Veronica and I would have to address two areas of her lifestyle that can dramatically impact exercise and nutrition but are very often overlooked: sleep and stress.

There are no hard and fast rules when it comes to initiating exercise, nutrition, and lifestyle changes. For some clients like Veronica, we knew focusing on her lifestyle factors made sense as a starting point because she didn't have the bandwidth to take on more right away. You may know your sleep or stress management could use improvement but still feel able to prioritize the exercise and nutrition "Big Rocks" at the same time.

You'll find that these three areas are all so interconnected that, regardless of where you choose to start, the other areas will benefit. Eating a more nutritious diet will help you sleep and handle stress better. It'll help you have more energy for your workouts. Working out will inspire you to want to eat for your goals and being active can relieve stress and help you fall asleep more quickly. Sleeping more will reduce food cravings and help you have more energy for your workout. You get the idea.

It's up to you if you want to address the "Big Rocks" in these chapters simultaneously or individually. You'll find that there's a lot of overlap between them, so your focus on one will naturally benefit the others. Don't stress about the best "order of operations" and give yourself permission to just start wherever makes the most sense for you. In my coaching program, we encourage setting one exercise, one nutrition, and one lifestyle goal each week (you'll learn more about goal setting in Part 3).

Being stressed or under-rested can make the difference between waking up for your morning workout or hitting snooze. Going for a walk after dinner or diving head first into the pantry. Being able to stop when you're satisfied or continuing to eat just because it's there. Making it through the "grind" or giving up in the midst of it.

Unfortunately, maintaining high stress levels and getting minimal sleep are two areas much of our culture seems to glorify. As a result, it's easy to wear them as a badge of honor and neglect their importance.

In reality, prioritizing these lifestyle factors can make consistently hitting your exercise and nutrition "Big Rocks" so much easier, not to mention dramatically improve nearly all areas of your life

Next, we'll review each one in depth, and I'll offer tips on how to improve them.

Why Sleep Matters

I'm sure you know that sleep is important, but you may not realize just *how* important it is! Lack of sleep is linked to all sorts of negative consequences, like:

- increased rates of depression[6]
- increased dementia risk[7]

---

[6] https://www.ncbi.nlm.nih.gov/pmc/articles/PMC4318605/
[7] https://www.nih.gov/news-events/nih-research-matters/lack-sleep-middle-age-may-increase-dementia-risk

- increased inflammation[8]

- muscle loss (for example, in one study[9], participants underwent the same caloric restriction, but the sleep deprived group lost less fat and more muscle)

- higher caloric intake[10] (due to both hormonal changes and having more awake but inactive time in which to eat)

- decreased self-control and decision-making abilities[11]

- decreased immune system function[12]

- increased risk of heart disease and stroke[13]

- fatigue and lack of motivation[14] and desire to exercise

Ghrelin, a hormone released by the stomach to signal hunger in the brain, is increased by about 15% when you're sleep deprived, while leptin, a hormone released by fat cells to indicate fullness to the brain, is decreased by about 15%. Cortisol, a stress hormone that can increase appetite is also increased when sleep deprived. Insulin, a hormone that moves sugar from the bloodstream to use for energy, may be produced in higher amounts when sleep deprived to combat resistance to it (more sugar staying in the bloodstream, so more insulin

---

[8] https://www.health.harvard.edu/sleep/how-sleep-deprivation-can-cause-inflammation
[9] https://pubmed.ncbi.nlm.nih.gov/20921542/
[10] https://www.ncbi.nlm.nih.gov/pmc/articles/PMC3763921/
[11] https://neuroptimal.com/wp-content/uploads/2019/05/sleep-deprivation.pdf
[12] https://www.cdc.gov/niosh/work-hour-training-for-nurses/longhours/mod2/05.html
[13] https://www.ncbi.nlm.nih.gov/pmc/articles/PMC2845795/
[14] https://www.dovepress.com/sleep-restriction-reduces-cognitive-but-not-physical-motivation-peer-reviewed-fulltext-article-NSS

produced to try to move it). This can increase hunger, body fat storage, and be a precursor for type 2 diabetes.

The result of all these hormonal changes is you being hungrier, having more cravings for highly palatable foods like chips and sweets, and being less satisfied when you do eat.

Suffice it to say, lack of sleep makes losing weight and keeping it off that much more difficult.

Although it might seem like there's nothing we can do to get more sleep—there is! Of course, there are some periods in your life when getting enough restful sleep just isn't an option, like when you have a newborn at home. Outside of those times, which are temporary and for good reason, making sleep a priority will help you lose weight and live a generally healthy lifestyle. You don't need to continue dragging through the day surviving on coffee and energy drinks, and if you want to lose weight, your lack of sleep could well be part of what's holding you back from seeing results.

Many of us resist going to bed earlier because we feel compelled to tidy the house first, we want to check our work emails one more time, or it feels like those late-night hours are the only ones we have for ourselves. We engage in "revenge bedtime procrastination" wherein we choose to sacrifice sleep for leisure time, not realizing its negative impacts.

All that to say, just about everything is easier and better when you're well rested. It's not an afterthought or "nice to have," or for the weak, lazy, or dead; it's an essential priority.

Fortunately, there are some simple routines and lifestyle habits you can implement to help you prioritize getting in seven-plus hours of restful sleep most nights. If you already do these consistently and still have trouble falling or staying asleep, ask your doctor if you would benefit from a sleep study to help pinpoint underlying health issues that could be contributing.

To improve sleep:

- stick to a schedule with regular wake and sleep times
- have a relaxing nighttime ritual
- sleep in a cold, dark, quiet environment (no TV or screens!)
- avoid alcohol and caffeine later in the day
- keep a journal by your bed to "brain dump" your To Do's or any thoughts swirling around in your head (i.e., writing down everything and anything that comes to your mind)
- listen to a sleep meditation or sleep-inducing podcast
- if you can't sleep, get out of bed and do something relaxing in another room until you feel tired

Veronica and I approached these changes gradually to ensure they would last and she would be sleeping a more optimal amount long term, not just for a few weeks. She elected to start by eliminating weekday alcohol, since she knew that would have a huge impact not just on her quality of sleep but also cut down on excess calories (both from the wine and the snacks she'd eat after a couple glasses). After a few weeks of working on her alcohol intake, she enacted a firm "no work after midnight" rule that allowed her to settle down hours earlier than she had been. When she realized that her thoughts were swirling after she'd turn off the light, she added nightly "brain dump" journaling and sleep meditations to her routine. These two to three extra hours of more restful sleep carried over into her waking hours, making it easier for her to get up in the morning, improving her mood, reducing her cravings, and reducing her need for caffeine during the day. Instead of feeling stuck, she felt energetic, happier, and more alive.

You can expect to experience a similar ripple effect of benefits when you choose to make small and gradual lifestyle changes to make sleep a priority, as well. You'll be happier, have more energy, find it easier to stay committed to your goals, and the weight will come off more easily, too! The following questions will help you assess and, if necessary, improve your current sleep habits.

Sleep Considerations & Next Steps

Are you currently getting at least seven hours of sleep per night? If not, how many hours do you typically get?

How long does it take you to fall asleep?

Based on the time you need to wake up, what is your ideal bedtime to ensure you're getting seven or more hours of sleep per night? What time does this mean getting into bed? Starting to wind down?

If you've determined that your sleep habits could use improvement, which of the suggestions from this section feel like a good place to start?

Why Stress Matters

Veronica felt like her stress was inevitable—and some of it was, like the occasions she was working under a tight deadline! But *how much* stress she experienced on a regular basis, how she thought about it, and the strategies she used to cope (like stress eating) made a big difference in her health, happiness, and ability to lose weight.

Like not getting enough sleep, having high levels of chronic stress also causes hormonal fluctuations that negatively impact hunger, satiety, fat storage, and fat breakdown.

The stressors our ancestors faced, like running away from a predator, were intense but short-lived. Our body's fight-or-flight response makes sense when you think about needing immediate resources to avoid being dinner for a saber-toothed tiger:

- Cortisol is released
- Glucose (stored carbs) flood the bloodstream to be used to for energy
- Insulin production is halted so the glucose can be used immediately
- Blood pumps harder and faster due to arteries narrowing and heart rate increasing
- Stressor is resolved (you survived!)
- Cortisol and other hormones return to normal

The problem with *modern* day stressors is that they're chronic, rather than acute. As a result, our cortisol levels are also chronically elevated. Cortisol suppresses insulin (the hormone that moves glucose *from* the bloodstream), which means that the glucose being consistently released *into* the bloodstream never actually makes it to the cells for energy. This combination results in energy-starved cells that want glucose they're not getting. Their response? Send hunger signals to the brain. As such, our appetites increase when we're chronically stressed and we're more likely to crave (and overeat) high-calorie foods. (In addition, for many of us, food is offered for comfort from an early age, so eating to avoid feeling our emotions can feel like an automatic reaction. This emotional eating also contributes to excess calories.)

Chronically elevated cortisol may also be linked to insomnia, dementia, depression, thyroid disorders, compromised digestion and absorption of food, and disrupted production of sex hormones.[15]

Like lack of sleep, chronic stress can also cause inflammation, and in an effort to reduce it, our bodies keep cortisol levels high. Over time, this can suppress our immune systems, which can lead to a whole host of consequences such as increased risk of GI issues, food allergies, autoimmune diseases, and cancer.

Although all this may sound scary, there's a lot we can do to reduce inflammation and stress, which will lower cortisol, decrease our risk of disease, and improve our overall health. The goal is not to eliminate stress entirely, but to reduce unnecessary stressors and learn how to navigate them without turning to counterproductive behaviors like alcohol and emotional eating.

One way Veronica and I worked to reduce her stress was to practice reframing her day-to-day responsibilities as opportunities to live by her values (more on this in Chapter

---

[15] https://www.ncbi.nlm.nih.gov/pmc/articles/PMC6371989

10), rather than as time-consuming tasks she "had" to do. Of course, not *everything* that causes stress needs to be framed in a positive light. Some life stuff just sucks. But for the more mundane of our stressors, for example, shuttling kids to after-school activities, we can choose how we think about them, and it can make a big difference in how we feel about them!

When it comes to chauffeuring our kids around, many of us resent the disruptions to our schedules or time spent stuck in traffic. Veronica did, too, until we started talking about ways to reduce her overall stress, and she decided to focus on being grateful for having healthy and active children and the conversations facilitated by being in the car together.

As she worked on making this mental switch, she found that instead of pick-ups and drop-offs feeling like more items on her never-ending To Do list, she actually looked forward to those reprieves from the workday to reconnect with her family and be present as a mom. Once *she* stopped acting so put out, she noticed her kids would let down their guards and often shared more about their lives on those car rides than at any other time. A task she had once resented turned into one of her favorite parts of the day and no longer felt like it was contributing to her stress.

Just like sleep can improve exercise and nutrition, and exercise and nutrition can improve sleep, the same goes for managing stress. Things like prioritizing nutritious foods that support weight loss and overall health (coming up in Chapter 8), minimizing caffeine and alcohol, learning to set and uphold boundaries (see Chapter 13), and working on overcoming your all-or-nothing patterns, will all help you learn to manage stress—and lose weight! You can't go wrong no matter where you start, and starting *anywhere* will help you make improvements all around!

Veronica had already made great progress on the caffeine and alcohol fronts when we focused on sleep, so she felt that a useful next step would be to set aside an hour or so on Sundays to prepare breakfasts and lunches for herself for the work week. She knew her habit of only having coffee until midafternoon was exacerbating her stress and late-night eating. Now that she was better rested, she felt ready to set a nutrition goal, especially one she knew would *also* support her goal of reducing stress!

She was shocked at the big impact these small changes were having on her cravings—they were almost completely gone! (This was due to a variety of factors: fueling herself better throughout the day, developing better coping mechanisms to recognize and process her emotions, reducing overall stress so her hunger and fullness hormones weren't out of whack, and breaking the habit of nighttime snacking).

It's important to be able to recognize the signs of feeling stressed and overwhelmed and be intentional about stopping to recharge throughout the day rather than letting your battery drain until you have nothing left to give. Developing more robust coping skills like learning to pause, notice and name your emotions, reflect on them, and then make mindful, intentional decisions, will help you deal with stress without instinctively turning to food, alcohol, or other counterproductive behaviors.

Veronica learned that when she got overwhelmed, her face feeling flushed and a heaviness in her chest, the stress ball her doctor had given her after she left the hospital wasn't enough. She practiced taking a few deep breaths, saying out loud, "I'm feeling really overwhelmed right now," and getting away from her desk for a few minutes to walk, stretch, get fresh air, or do a five-minute meditation.

At night when she felt the pantry calling her name, she wouldn't act on the feeling right away but would pause and remind herself that she wasn't physically hungry and that food wasn't going to lessen her workload. She got in the habit of brushing her teeth after dinner so she would feel like she was done eating for the day and prioritizing her nighttime to do's to help address the overwhelm and take productive action.

As Veronica addressed the day-to-day stress, she recognized the need to set some boundaries at work, like not checking her email after she logged out for the day, and improve her time management skills, both of which helped her reduce her stress levels and free up more time for herself, exercise, hobbies, and friendships that helped her feel fulfilled.

Here are some common strategies that have helped my clients manage their stress so it doesn't hinder their weight-loss efforts. It's not a comprehensive list but will give you some ideas for where to start:

- Spend time outdoors
- Meditate
- Try acupuncture
- Get a new hobby you enjoy
- Start or end your day with journaling
- Express gratitude more often
- Develop a yoga practice
- Reach out to friends
- Laugh more often
- Do breathwork
- Take walks

Don't worry if you have a lot of stress right now that you're not sure how to mitigate. Like Veronica, you can make one small change at a time and trust that those will add up and have a big impact! The coming chapters will help you increase your skills and confidence to be successful long term. Working with a mental health professional can also help you learn how to navigate the stress in your life in healthier and more productive ways.

Stress Considerations and Next Steps

On a scale of 1-10, how would you rate your current levels of chronic stress?

What do you currently do to manage or cope with stress? Do you engage in any self-sabotaging behaviors that you can connect to stress?

What would you like to be different about your stress levels and/or how you handle stress?

What new coping mechanisms would you like to learn or develop to help you reduce stress?

What is one strategy that feels the most feasible to implement this week?

Because exercise, lifestyle, and nutrition are so intertwined, fueling your body with nutritious foods that support weight loss and general health will help you have more energy, see better results from your workouts, sleep better, reduce chronic inflammation, and feel better equipped to handle life's stressors. It's time to learn the nutrition "Big Rocks"!

CHAPTER 8

NUTRITION "BIG ROCKS"

Tanya begrudgingly peeled the plastic off today's Lean Cuisine. Swedish Meatballs. Actually one of her favorites, but after eating these meals for eight months of lunches during the workweek, none of them were super appealing.

But between those and the fact that she'd started intermittent fasting instead of eating breakfast, she was eating way less overall. Sure, she'd been hungry a lot, but she felt like it was worth it, at least while the scale had been moving!

Now that the scale *wasn't* moving—and she'd had hundreds of meals like these—she was starting to resent them. She was ravenous by the time lunch rolled around, and the microwave meals seemed like they were making her hungrier, rather than satisfying her.

Back in the winter and spring, Tanya would just chew gum and go to bed early when she started to feel snacky. But now, all bets were off. She felt burnt out from being so restrictive and found herself only able to be "good" for a few days before she binged on these amazing cookies from the bakery down the street.

Once she "blew it" for the day or weekend, she would just keep eating. She ate out of frustration that the scale wasn't moving the way she wanted it to, and if she was working so hard and eating so little but had nothing to show for it, why even bother?

Tanya's lack of focus on the exercise "Big Rocks" weren't the only reasons she was feeling so crappy and had stopped seeing progress. She was also overlooking the nutrition "Big Rocks" and instead was alternating between eating very little and binging (another example of all-or-nothing behavior), designating foods as "good" or "bad," and stressing over "Pebbles" like her fasting window.

In the previous chapter, we covered the four ways our body *burns* calories:

- Basal metabolic rate (BMR) (staying alive calories)
- Thermic effect of food (TEF) (digestive calories)
- Exercise activity thermogenesis (EAT) (exercise calories)
- Non-exercise activity thermogenesis (NEAT) (daily movement calories)

Calories going out is only one side of the energy balance equation, so before I tell you the nutrition "Big Rocks," let's talk about the calories coming in (much more straightforward).

Calories in come from two places: food and drinks

You'll remember from the previous chapter that in order to lose weight, you must be in a **caloric deficit**, or take in fewer calories than your body uses throughout the day. This negative energy balance is essential for fat loss and the reason that every single diet works, even if the focus isn't on the calories.

Total Calories out > Total Calories in = Weight Loss

When Tanya started her nothing-but-Lean-Cuisine diet, she drastically reduced the number of calories she was taking in (and increased the number of calories she was expending due to her new workout routine). This created a pretty significant deficit.

We covered one of the reasons her weight loss started to plateau in the previous chapter: now that there was less of her, her BMR—and therefore her calorie needs—was lower.

The other reason, the one she was currently overlooking, was the fact that increasingly frequent binges were adding hundreds of calories to her day and bumping her out of the deficit she was certain she was still in.

It's very easy to focus on the choices we're making that are aligned with our goals and overlook or minimize the frequency of choices we make that aren't. I'll talk more about the importance of overcoming this disconnect in a bit, but for now, back to caloric deficits.

Since being in a deficit means not taking in as much energy as your body needs, it will break down whatever is available (glucose from carbs, amino acids from protein/muscle tissue, and fatty acids from body fat) to support necessary bodily functions.

Your goal is to maximize *fat* burning while minimizing muscle breakdown *and* prioritizing your overall health. So, the nutrition "Big Rocks" are:

1. Calories
2. Protein
3. Fiber

Learning what the right amounts of these things are for YOU, what foods contain them, how to prioritize them most of the time while also including your favorite foods that you just enjoy, even if they're not particularly nutritious, helps you put yourself in a position where you can maintain a healthy weight without thinking about food all the time.

When you keep it simple and just focus on these "Big Rocks," you free up more energy to identify and overcome the obstacles that prevent you from doing them consistently and get out of that "I know what to do but I'm just not doing it" cycle. Let's go over each one.

Nutrition Big Rock #1: Calories

Since a negative calorie balance (caloric deficit) is what drives weight loss, calories are king and how many you're taking in matters, whether you like it or not.

Most diets you've tried in the past that haven't utilized food tracking as a tool have created a deficit without putting the emphasis on calories, either through selling you low-calorie packaged meals and snacks, asking you to eliminate certain foods or groups, giving you a fasting window, or replacing meals with lower-calorie liquid feedings. At the end of the day, it wasn't the length of your fasting window or anything special in your shakes that caused the weight loss: you were just taking in fewer calories without realizing it.

Tanya, like many women, was making several crucial mistakes when it came to calories. Initially, she had slashed calories way too low; in a way, the frustrations she was feeling were inevitable. Motivation is generally high when you start a new weight-loss attempt, so it's easier to white-knuckle through something that is actually pretty unsustainable, especially when you feel like the result is worth the sacrifice. Inevitably motivation wanes, though, and initial results often taper, the combination of which threatens consistency and, ultimately, your success.

Although it might feel like the bigger calorie deficit, the better, that's just not the case.

Although it's appealing to want to lose weight as quickly as possible, it's actually not good for you in the short or long term (exceptions may apply in extreme situations, in which case, please see your doctor).

Restricting calories too much can lead to malnutrition, which can cause a whole cascade of negative consequences from extreme fatigue to brittle nails, hair loss, a compromised immune system, weakened bones, and osteoporosis. Drastically undereating for an extended period of time can also cause dehydration, gallstones, muscle loss (more on that in the next section), and an increased likelihood of regaining the weight.

Tanya didn't understand why she was able to stick to her plan so well before but now felt it impossible. She blamed her lack of willpower or discipline and was getting increasingly mad at herself. She wasn't making the connection between eating so little during the day and her nearly-impossible-to-ignore cravings later.

Even though she was frustrated that she was eating so many unplanned cookies, she wasn't thinking about how many extra calories she was taking in during her binges and still felt like she was eating very little, at least most of the time. She wasn't able to zoom out and look at the big picture, which would have revealed to her that despite feeling like she was eating so little, she was actually taking in more calories than she realized.

Tanya's experience highlights the other risks of cutting calories too low: being unable to consistently eat so little, binging on "bad" foods, not seeing results, getting the worst of both worlds (being hungry a lot AND feeling uncomfortably full a lot), and the risk of giving up out of frustration and gaining the weight back.

How many calories **you** need depends on a lot of factors, and it's important to remember that no equation or calculation can give you anything more than an estimated starting point.

[**Note:** Inside your book portal is a calculator you can use to estimate your own needs. The following explanation is just so you understand what information goes into this equation. I would recommend waiting to calculate your targets until you have read this section and the sections on protein and fiber.]

Of the available equations, Mifflin-St Jeor is the most accurate (this is the one used in the book portal), found to estimate within 10% of a person's TDEE for 82% of people. (As you can see, there's still a decent margin of error there).

Equations like these take your age, height, and weight into account, all of which are knowable variables with minimal room for error. The variable with the biggest margin in the equation is your activity level.

Just as we have a tendency to underestimate how many calories are coming in, humans also have a tendency to overestimate how many are going out. We tend to focus on how many calories we burn during our workouts and overlook how sedentary we are the rest of the day.

Keep in mind that all people are on the same spectrum of activity. If soldiers are on their feet all day, carrying 50-plus pounds of gear, and Olympic athletes have multiple-hours-long training sessions, where does that leave us mere mortals? Probably closer to the sedentary or lightly active end of the spectrum than the extremely active end.

Here are some general criteria you can use to help decide on the most appropriate activity level for your current lifestyle:

Sedentary—Mostly under ~6,000 steps/day, largely sedentary job, sporadic or no workouts, sedentary hobbies outside of work

Lightly Active—Mostly over ~6,000 steps/day, to to three workouts per week that are usually under an hour, job that requires or allows for some movement throughout the day, occasionally engaging in somewhat active hobbies. (Or some combination of these).

Moderately Active—Consistently over ~8,000 steps/day, three to five 30- to 90-minute workouts per week, consistent movement throughout the day during and outside of work.

Highly Active—Consistently over ~10,000 steps/day, 60-plus minute workouts most days of the week, strenuous job and/or hobbies

Extremely Active—Consistently over ~15,000 steps/day, 60-plus minute workouts most days of the week, very strenuous jobs and/or hobbies (athletes, constantly moving heavy things at work, etc.)

The purpose of estimating your activity level is to estimate your total calorie needs and give yourself a starting point for how many calories you'll likely need to eat in order to lose weight. You needn't stress about exactly where you fall on the activity spectrum, and if you are torn between two multipliers, I would recommend calculating your TDEE with both and starting somewhere in the middle. (Remember, all you're getting here is a starting point, not a number that's set in stone!)

The steps in your book portal will help you determine both your estimated TDEE and calorie target based on a 5-15% deficit. I do not recommend more than 15%, especially to start, because of the aforementioned.

Nutrition Big Rock #2: Protein

Lanie became a client after losing a significant amount of weight following the WW program. Prior to starting, she'd told herself that her constant lack of energy and recurring headaches must be related to the extra weight she was carrying around and would resolve once she'd dropped it.

Unfortunately, instead of feeling better with every pound lost, she was feeling just as bad—if not worse! After reaching her goal and still struggling to get through the day, she contacted me for help.

Within weeks of switching from counting points to tracking calories, protein, and fiber, her headaches had resolved and her energy was through the roof!

While calories are king when it comes to weight loss, losing weight doesn't necessarily mean improving your health. The other nutrition "Big Rocks," protein and fiber, help ensure that you feel satiated, energized, and properly nourished by eating a nutritious diet with plenty of important vitamins and minerals to maximize your overall health and quality of life.

There are a few reasons why protein is so important:

Protein is the most satiating of the macronutrients (protein, carbs, fat), which means when you eat it throughout the day, you're likely to be less hungry than if you were eating the same calories from other macros. This is especially helpful when you're in a caloric deficit and taking in fewer calories than you're used to. *Some* hunger may be inevitable, but you shouldn't be feeling super hungry all the time, and taking in sufficient protein can help ensure that you're not.

Protein helps you retain muscle while losing *fat*, which is how you change the shape, look, and feel of your body. Being in a caloric deficit, following a progressive strength-training program, and prioritizing protein are key to ensure you are losing fat while sacrificing as little muscle as possible (a little bit is inevitable and nothing to be concerned about).

Digesting protein burns more calories. Remember the thermic effect of food (TEF) from the last chapter? It takes more energy (aka calories) to digest and absorb protein than it does carbs and fat. (This doesn't add up to a substantial amount but is a nice bonus).

For these reasons combined, protein is our next nutrition "Big Rock."

So how much protein should you be eating?

The Recommended Daily Allowance (RDA) for protein is only .36g per pound of body weight (so just over

50g for a woman weighing 150 pounds), but the goal of an RDA is to avoid deficiency and doesn't necessarily suggest an optimal amount, especially for active adults looking to drop body fat.

Barring any health conditions for which your doctor suggests otherwise, the ideal range is much higher than the RDA, to the tune of around .5-1g per pound of body weight.[16]

If you are significantly overweight or obese, aim for the lower end of that range, or about .5-.7 grams of protein per pound of body weight.

If you are already fairly lean and looking to drop a little more fat, aim for the higher end of that range, or about .7-1 gram of protein per pound of body weight.

More protein is fine but not necessary or additionally beneficial, and it will likely just take away from a well-balanced diet with a variety of macro and micronutrients.

When you calculate these numbers (remember you can use the resources in the book portal to do the heavy lifting for you), you may be alarmed at how high they seem. Don't let this overwhelm you.

Just like we talked about with your step goal, it's fine if it takes some time to get yourself to where you want to be. First find your baseline, or the amount of protein you're currently averaging per day, then work on gradually increasing over the next several weeks or months. I'd start first with incremental goals.

For example, say you weigh 150 pounds, so you're aiming for 105g of protein per day (.7g/lb). Right now you eat around

---

[16] https://examine.com/guides/protein-intake/

70g on a typical day. Shoot for 80g for the next one or two weeks, then increase to 90g, and so on until you are consistently at your goal.

The easiest way to increase your protein is to look back at the foods you're already eating that are high in it and have a little more of them. Another option is to combine sources in one meal, for example adding ham to your scrambled eggs.

Swapping snacks for higher protein options like Greek yogurt and jerky can help, as well as other simple swaps like trying edamame or chickpea-based pasta instead of wheat and using bone broth instead of regular.

You can also consider adding in a protein bar or shake to supplement what you're already getting from whole food sources. I recommend limiting those to one serving per day so that the majority of your daily calories are coming from less processed, more nutrient-dense options, but they're convenient to have on hand when you need them or to serve as a stopgap while you work on increasing your protein in other ways.

Making protein a priority and working *toward* this range is better than not focusing on it at all.

Nutrition Big Rock #3: Fiber

I consider fiber to be the "final frontier" when it comes to nutrition. It's the target most women have the hardest time hitting consistently. (Protein usually takes the brunt of people's frustrations, but that's because most people aren't paying attention to fiber).

Fiber is a "Big Rock" because with the Gone For Good formula, you're not just losing weight. You're doing so while *also* prioritizing your overall health, rather than sacrificing the latter for the former.

Prioritizing fiber intake (a type of carbohydrate that passes through the body undigested) helps ensure that you're eating nutrient-dense foods and not just low-calorie, highly processed foods that help you hit your other "Big Rocks" but result in a mostly nutrient-void diet.

Regular bowel movements, one of fiber's most known benefits, isn't the only reason it's important. Fiber can also help lower cholesterol, blood pressure, and inflammation, help prevent diabetes (and improve blood sugar levels for people who already have it), and help with feeling satiated after meals.

I generally find it to be a good proxy marker for eating a diet with plenty of whole (unprocessed) foods that are rich in a variety of important vitamins and minerals.

The recommended fiber intake for women is 14 grams per 1,000 calories, which is generally in the range of 21-25 grams per day, yet the average North American eats less than 15g/day!

Like with your steps and protein, start where you are and gradually increase your fiber intake over time. In general, fruits, veggies, whole grains, and legumes are great sources of fiber, so work on adding more servings of those foods to your meals and you'll be getting more fiber and having higher volume meals that feel more satiating.

If you're feeling at all overwhelmed by trying to learn and master all of the nutrition "Big Rocks," focus first on your total calories, then increase your protein, and wait to tackle fiber until you're feeling more confident.

A Note about Carbs and Fats

You might be wondering about carbs and fat and how much of those you should be eating. Carbs are our bodies' preferred energy source, and fats are important for hormonal health, among other reasons, but at the end of the day, the exact amounts of them or ratio between them is much less important for fat loss, so they're Pebbles rather than the "Big Rocks."

I recommend hitting your calorie, protein, and fiber goals and letting your carbs and fat fall where they may. Once you've mastered the "Big Rocks," feel free to experiment with higher or lower amounts of each to see what makes YOU feel your best but as far as weight loss goes, that's not a top priority.

Nutrition Big Rocks Overview

Eating a nutritious diet is incredibly important for overall health, energy, and maintaining your ideal weight (even more so than exercise, largely because of how much easier it is to take *in* calories than it is to burn them!). It doesn't need to be confusing or time consuming. Keeping it simple and focusing on the "Big Rocks" of calories, protein, and fiber allows you to develop habits that make eating for your health goals as easy as possible, while freeing up more mental energy on overcoming the challenges.

Focus on:

1. Big Rock #1—Eating the right number of calories for your goals (a 5-15% deficit from your estimated total daily energy expenditure)

2. Big Rock #2—Prioritizing protein to help with satiety and muscle retention (~.7g/lb body weight spread across the day, ideally from whole food sources)

3. Big Rock #3—Prioritizing fiber to help with satiety and eating a nutritious diet that supports overall health, not just weight loss (20-plus g/day)

4. Pebble—Prioritizing foods that are high in volume (take up lots of space on a plate and in your stomach) to help reduce hunger and increase satiety.

5. Pebble—Once you feel like you have a strong grasp on the Big Rocks, feel free to experiment with less impactful things like carb/fat ratios, fasting/feeding windows, meal timing, etc. These aren't the primary drivers of weight loss but can help being in a deficit feel more sustainable and help you learn about what works best for your body.

A Note For Perimenopausal & Menopausal Women

Recent research has suggested that our metabolisms are actually pretty stable into our 60s, and it's lifestyle factors like eating more and moving less in subtle ways that contribute to the majority of the weight we gain with age.[17]

The hormonal fluctuations during perimenopause, and consistently low levels of those hormones in menopause, don't *cause* fat gain so much as they contribute to a whole host of unpleasant symptoms, like how your body

---

[17] https://www.science.org/doi/10.1126/science.abe5017

processes certain foods and changes to hunger and satiety, temperature regulation, mood, and more. These changes then impact everything from how much you're eating and moving to how well you're sleeping.

Body fat stores shift as you go through menopause, and you may notice your midsection looking thicker. Female bodies become more sensitive to carbs, so it may be beneficial to reduce starchy carbs except for before and/or after hard workouts. This does not mean you need to eat *low* carb, just that being more strategic with carb timing (once you learn to hit your "Big Rock" habits consistently) may be beneficial for reducing belly fat. At other meals, eat plenty of fibrous veggies that will provide lots of micronutrients, volume, and fiber, all of which will help with satiety.

A Note On Alcohol

No, you don't need to give up drinking. But you do need to know that whatever amount you're drinking is probably having a bigger negative impact on your results than you realize.

Despite what you might read in the media, such as sensationalized headlines about the health benefits of wine, no amount is considered healthy, and the cascade effect that a serving or two of alcohol can have on SO many of your body's processes is pretty overwhelming.

Just a couple examples include lowered inhibitions that lead to eating and drinking more than normal, less restful sleep, and the way the next day's hangover impacts your activity level and nutrition choices.

If you've been thinking about your consumption (or *know* it's having a negative impact), I strongly encourage you to consider reducing your intake to whatever amount you feel is worth the tradeoff in other areas of your life.

Establishing Your Baseline for the Exercise & Nutrition "Big Rocks"

For each "Big Rock," I recommend taking a similar approach: start where you are, compare that to where you want to be, and gradually adjust to get there in a way that feels sustainable and eventually becomes your lifestyle.

Figuring out where you are now can sometimes be easier said than done. Most of us have a major lack of awareness of what we're actually doing on a day-to-day basis.

We have selective memories and tend to focus on the behaviors that support our goals while overlooking the ones that *don't* (which add up more quickly than we think).

When it comes to exercise, that looks like telling ourselves that we're "pretty active" when, in reality, we get in sporadic workouts and only walk the dog when he whines. Or we work out hard and consistently but feel like that checks the movement box, so we only walk a few thousand steps outside of that.

When it comes to nutrition, it looks like telling ourselves that we eat "pretty healthy" when, in reality, we're overlooking the hundreds of calories we eat and drink most days outside of mealtimes or unrelated to true physical hunger. (Like the wine you can't open fast enough after a stressful day or the chips on the couch while catching up with a friend).

Without the awareness of what you're *currently* doing, it's very hard to know what has to change in order to lose weight. It's like trying to get directions on your phone but not knowing where you're starting from.

As such, the first step toward learning and mastering the exercise and nutrition "Big Rocks" is tracking them to develop this objective awareness.

Tracking Your Exercise "Big Rocks"

Establishing your exercise baseline is fairly straightforward: print a blank calendar or use one you already have in your planner or on the wall. At the end of the day, jot down your total steps or active time, whether you took a rest/recovery day or worked out (and, if so, whether you did strength, cardio, or another form of exercise).

After a few weeks, you'll have a much better handle on your typical movement and how to start getting closer to the weekly routine laid out in the previous chapter.

For example, you may see that you're averaging one to two strength workouts per week and know that you want to work on increasing that until you're consistently getting in three. You may realize that you are taking 9,000-plus steps on weekdays but are only taking around 3,000 on weekends, so you'll want to make more of an intentional effort to walk on those days.

Tracking Your Nutrition "Big Rocks"

The nutrition "Big Rocks" are a little more time consuming to track and may require learning a new skill, but it's well worth the effort.

While the act of food tracking can be polarizing, I think such a reaction is unwarranted. Documenting what you're eating is an incredibly useful tool for developing the awareness I keep harping on. That awareness is what gives you the *opportunity* to start making different choices that better support your goals and the lasting weight loss you're after.

If you've attempted to track your food or count calories/macros in the past and had a negative experience with it, it's likely for one of a few reasons. You were:

- struggling to learn something new and be a beginner at something you weren't naturally good at right away

- trying to be perfect (hitting your targets on the nose every day)

- stressing yourself out over "macro tetris" (trying to hit a calorie, protein, carb, fiber, and fat target all at the same time)

- viewing it as a chore that you *had* to do rather than a useful tool that would help you reach the weight loss goal that YOU care about

- you don't want to be confronted with, or take ownership of, the choices you're making once you're aware of them

Tracking isn't to blame for any of those things, and that doesn't have to be your experience in the future.

Imagine you want to start saving more money. How would you start?

Maybe you already know you spend way too much at Target, so you stop going there so often. That might work but you may still not be saving as much as you'd like. Then what?

Taking a look at your bank statement would help you get crystal clear on how much money is coming in, how much is going out, and where it's going. Though you might be surprised or embarrassed by what you learn, the bank statement itself isn't *causing* you to feel that way.

The bank statement is neutral. It's just a reflection of where your money has always been going. The difference now is that you're aware of it, and it's highlighted some changes you can make if you're serious about your savings goal.

Tracking can help you:

- better understand what portion sizes are appropriate for you
- learn the calorie content of your favorite foods
- stop categorizing foods as good or bad
- understand how to put together balanced meals that leave you feeling satiated and energized
- start to make choices more aligned with your goals just because you know you'll be documenting them

The goal is not to track your food forever. These and other intangible skills, like reconnecting with your hunger and fullness cues, learning to stop when you're satisfied, and developing the coping skills to manage your emotions without turning to food will help you maintain a healthy weight long term, *without* tracking (aka eating more intuitively).

You can decide, right now, that tracking your food for a while is something you *want* to do because it will help you be more successful at losing weight and keeping it off this time.

You can decide that the knowledge you learn and skills you develop are worth the discomfort of being a beginner at something new.

As with any tool, how long to use it varies depending on the circumstances, so I can't tell you exactly how long you should track, but I would recommend committing to a minimum of one week to understand your current baseline. From there, I think most women would benefit from tracking for a few months, after which point you may feel confident about stopping and continuing to lose weight or maintaining on your own. If tracking continues to feel like a useful tool beyond that, there's no need to stop before you're ready. When the time comes, ease yourself out of tracking so you can prove to yourself that the changes you've made will stick whether you're documenting them or not.

If you already *know*—even without tracking—which of your current habits (or lack thereof) aren't serving you, make a list of those and start tackling them in whatever order makes sense for you to ultimately focus on all six of the exercise and nutrition "Big Rocks."

If you're not sure why you're not losing weight because you feel like you're already doing everything right or eating very little, or you've already addressed the "low-hanging fruit" (easy-to-recognize areas of opportunity like mindless snacking and liquid calories), tracking is your most useful tool to determine the next habits to tackle.

If you're willing to give it a try, I would recommend downloading a free tracking app (MyFitnessPal is my preference) and committing to diligently tracking a week of eating and drinking as you normally do. This will help you understand how many calories and how much protein and fiber you're currently eating and how that compares to your needs for weight loss and overall health improvements. For greatest accuracy, use a food scale when possible to measure servings in grams or ounces. If that's impractical or not an option, using measuring cups and spoons or even just eyeballing portions still provide useful information.

When you look back at your log, you'll likely be able to see easy changes you can make to improve what you're currently doing, build some momentum, and help you start tackling the "Big Rocks."

Then it's just a matter of being consistent, learning as you go, and remembering that the real learning happens when you look back at your log and use that information to help you make the gradual changes necessary to reach your goal in a way that feels sustainable. This could be things like realizing that you eat more in the afternoons when you skip breakfast, that your favorite Starbucks drink is 300 calories, or that your "occasional" glass of wine is more like two glasses most nights.

If you have a lot of questions right now, that's normal. The best way to learn is by starting. And if you need help, we'll talk more about who to enlist in the next chapter.

For now, journaling on the following prompts will help you make sense of what to change and how to start.

Journaling Prompts

What Pebbles are you spending time and energy on?

What beliefs or behaviors are you willing to let go of to free up the time/energy to prioritize the "Big Rocks"?

CHAPTER 9

COMPREHENSIVE SUPPORT

Before working with a new client, I ask her to fill out a short application and have a phone call with me so we can make sure we're a good fit.

One of the questions I ask is what this woman is looking to get out of coaching. Here is a sampling of their responses:

- "I need you to listen, not just give me a statistical or book answer. We are all unique and I need out-of-the-box help that's made for ME."

- "I keep telling myself I can do it on my own but I haven't been 100% committed. I can do the counting/tracking on my own but I'm not. I'm finally admitting that I need help."

- "I need help untwisting the mess I have created in my head. I need to learn healthy habits that will work for myself (and my husband) for a lifetime."

- "To help me be okay with being imperfect. Get me on the right road to a simpler, easier way of life—with accountability. I want to be able to enjoy my life again. I don't want it to be so hard."

- "I want to be taught more and not feel like I am dieting for the rest of my life. I would love for a coach to help me with how I see myself and my body. I want to love my body."

- "Helping me know what to do, keep it simple, not complicate it. Point me in the right direction. Somebody who knows more than me."

- "I need help staying motivated when there are setbacks and someone to call me out when I am making excuses."

Asking For Help

I know asking for help isn't easy.

Several years ago, when I was first starting my business, I was too stubborn (prideful?) to ask for help. Instead, I spent hours reading blogs from online marketers who promised to reveal all their secrets if I just attended this free webinar.

For months I agonized over seemingly important decisions like logos and brand colors, wrote blogs no one would read, created freebies no one would download, and generally ran myself ragged doing all sorts of things that didn't matter.

I had exactly zero clients, prospects, or idea of what I was even selling. I spent countless evenings complaining to my incredibly supportive husband, Grey, that I was working so hard, doing everything I was supposed to be doing, and nothing was working! I knew I was qualified and capable but being my own boss sounded a lot cooler before I realized I had no idea what I was doing without some direction and accountability.

My husband suggested investing in my business—and myself—dozens of times before I finally listened (though I'm sure I thought it was my groundbreaking idea at the time!).

Admitting I needed help felt like admitting defeat. Like I wasn't good enough or smart enough to do it on my own and that meant I would *never* be good or smart enough.

That was more than eight years ago, and once I started investing financially in mentorship and community, I haven't stopped. All it took was one experienced and understanding coach to have me kicking myself for not asking for help sooner.

I came to realize that asking for help isn't a sign of weakness, at all, but a sign of strength. It takes courage to confide in someone that you're struggling on your own and could use a hand.

Importance Of Community

Part of why comprehensive support is so important is because of the fallout of feeling like you've tried and "failed" at losing weight so many times before. Each failure chips away at your confidence that you can be successful in the future and prevents you from even trying again! That self-doubt *has* to be addressed for you to keep the weight off this time.

Getting help isn't just about finding a capable mentor; most of us are most successful with a whole team of support around us.

Motivational speaker Jim Rohn is credited with saying, "You are the average of the five people you spend the most time with," a quote that has come to represent the importance of being intentional about the people with whom we surround ourselves, both to positively impact the likelihood of reaching our goals and to ward off the overwhelmingly negative health consequences of being lonely and socially isolated (which was recently deemed a public health issue because of its association with higher rates of heart disease, obesity, depression, anxiety, and dementia).

Comprehensive support comes not just in the form of mentorship but also community. Not just guidance from trusted professionals but also peers to learn from, teach, and connect with outside of a shared goal of losing weight.

Journal Prompts

Pause and write down the five to ten people you spend the most time with.

Are they default connections based on convenience or circumstance (coworkers you don't even like, relatives who don't "get" you?)

Of those relationships, who is most supportive of your weight-loss goals and you becoming the person you want to be?

Who is the least supportive?

How do they show/not show their support?

As I mentioned in Chapter 2, part of why keeping weight off long term is so difficult is because it most likely puts you in the minority among just about everyone you know. Unless you're intentional about curating your comprehensive support system, odds are, the people you're spending most of your time with *aren't* 100% supportive of your goals (though they might say they are).

When the goals of the people around you aren't aligned with yours, it's very easy to get pulled back to center by the **status quo bias,** or the preference for maintaining one's current situation and opposing actions that may change the state of affairs.

You don't want to stand out or rock the boat too much so you just go with the flow. Or you are easily peer pressured into doing things that are the norm among your group or might be fun in the moment but are at odds with your long-term goals and the person you want to be.

It's much easier to stay committed and take consistent action toward your goals when the people around you are in it with you. As you may have experienced, it's easier to focus on losing weight when all of your friends are also doing Dry January or are concerned about wearing bikinis on an upcoming beach vacation than it is at other times of the year when their priorities may be elsewhere.

It's important to be intentional about whose opinions you listen to and with whom you surround yourself so that you're inspired to learn, grow, evolve, and live your healthiest life, rather than being pulled back down to the status quo by those who don't want to change themselves.

With only a small minority (10-20%) of people who reach their weight-loss goals being able to maintain those results long term, and a high percentage (80%) having one or more health risks, unless you are very fortunate or have been intentional up until this point, the people around you right now are likely *not* the people you should be turning to for health advice. Here are some scary statistics about the health of American women: 44% are living with some form of heart disease (the leading cause of death for women over 40)[18] and 80% of women aged 40-60 have one or more risk for it.[19]

---

[18] https://www.cdc.gov/heartdisease/women.htm
[19] https://www.nhlbi.nih.gov/health/coronary-heart-disease/women

The unhealthy, unsustainable, short-term focused, "get this weight off at all costs—and fast!" approaches that most women take to lose weight come back to bite them when they lead to worsened health and the weight piling back on.

This cannot continue to be the approach you take if your goal is to be in good health and keep the weight off for the rest of your life.

Having health-minded friends and mentors, whether local to you or online, will help you maintain your weight loss by making healthy habits the norm and encouraging you to continue creating the body and life you really want, as opposed to getting comments about how you're already skinny enough and shouldn't "be obsessed" or how you should "live a little," as opposed to encouraging you to continue creating the body and life you really want.

The people we surround ourselves with extend more than ever to online platforms, which can take a huge toll on our ideas of "normal" or "ideal."

While social media has made it easier than ever to connect with like-minded individuals, we've also never been more vulnerable to the quacks out there with snake oil to sell. It can be hard to differentiate between qualified professionals and those preying on your insecurities. How many followers someone has is, unfortunately, a terrible indicator of the quality of the advice they give.

One giant red flag is when someone suggests that there's only *one* way to achieve an outcome (their way) and all others are wrong or dangerous.

As you know from the previous chapter, all weight loss is the result of being in a caloric deficit, but *how* you go about creating that deficit will vary from person to person and depends a lot on your lifestyle and personality.

A Note on Social Media

"The Socials" can be a double-edged sword that can either help you find your community or make you feel even more isolated and alone.

Before you finish this chapter, I challenge you to do a social media cleanse where you unfollow, mute, or remove any person or profile that makes you feel less than, whether it's due to the actual nature of their content or the feelings seeing their generally harmless content evokes in you.

I do this every six months or so to make sure that I'm not setting myself up for a doom spiral every time I log on.

Remember that YOU control your social media usage, not vice versa (though it can certainly feel that way).

Existing Friends & Family

There are several ways relationships can change as you pursue your weight-loss goals and begin stepping into the identity of a fit and healthy person.

Hopefully, the people closest to you will be encouraging and eventually inspired to make their own positive changes, and you all grow and evolve together.

I see this with clients who don't force any of their changes onto their spouses or friends, who just lead by example, who make the changes that support their health and happiness, and who let their results speak for themselves. This is exactly what happened with my client, Sally, and her family. Just learning and mastering the exercise and nutrition "Big Rocks" changed the food she bought, meals she prepared, and how she and her husband and friends spent time together. Her husband lost weight and improved his blood pressure, and she started meeting friends for walks instead of happy hours, a change everyone was happy with!

Another possibility is that the people around you *don't* get inspired to make a change and may even feel threatened by how the relationship dynamic changes as you become healthier, happier, and more confident.

Relationships that had a power imbalance to begin with may become even rockier.

It's rare that pursuing your health and weight-loss goals is the *sole* reason for a relationship to fall apart, but your personal growth may exacerbate the underlying issues and make them harder to ignore.

In this case, you may decide that you've outgrown the relationship and move on from it, rather than continuing to fight the downward pull from someone who doesn't want to lift themselves up.

Most relationships fall somewhere in the middle. Your friends or family aren't necessarily making their own (lasting) changes, but they're also not actively dissuading you from making them and may be happy to support you. These dynamics are likely to still shift over time, especially as you find new relationships that may be better aligned with the lifestyle you're creating.

This might look like seeing a friend less frequently or having firmer boundaries around where you go, what you do, or what you're comfortable talking about. My client Nat experienced this with her mom, whose weight had yo-yoed up and down for Nat's whole life and who resented the fact that Nat had broken the cycle and lost weight in a way she could keep off for good. She didn't understand Nat's boundary around not wanting to talk about their bodies, but it was something Nat knew she had to do in order to protect her mental health.

It's perfectly fine to set these boundaries and limitations around relationships that you don't want to give up but also know can't continue the way they have been earlier in your life.

In general, friends and family members typically make terrible accountability partners.

Most people close to you are either struggling with the same challenges you are or don't want to jeopardize the friendship by *actually* holding you accountable.

Think about it: you can *tell* your husband to call you out next time you show up on the couch with wine and cookies, but is he going to? (Probably not if he wants to have a pleasant evening or have a chance of getting some hanky-panky). Would you actually *want* him to? (Probably not). How are you going to react if he did? (Probably not by offering up some hanky-panky!)

What about your coworker? Do you really want her commenting on your lunch every day or whether you should be having that croissant? Encouraging you to hit your step goal but backhandedly bragging about how much farther she's walked?

The people in close proximity to us may not be the most appropriate to hold us accountable, but they can still help in other ways. To make sure the people in your life who are willing to help actually *are*, be direct and specific about what you need and also what you *don't* want; don't expect them to be able to read your mind.

If you want your spouse to stop bringing home wine when you say you've had a long day, TELL THEM and uphold the boundary when it happens.

If you want your kids to give you 20 minutes to get a workout in, TELL THEM and uphold the boundary when it happens.

If you're asking a coworker to help you keep your weight-loss goals at top of mind during all the hours you spend together at work, be specific about what you mean by that and exactly what you're looking for.

If friends, family, and coworkers aren't the best people to provide professional guidance and accountability on your weight-loss journey, who is?

Someone whose primary role in your life is to help you reach your goals, like a coach or a support group where other relationship dynamics don't threaten to distract from the task at hand: making sure you get the weight off and keep it off!

Board of Advisors

One of the best ways to rebuild your belief in yourself is to surround yourself with people who see your worth and know that you inherently have what it takes to be successful. There is something SO powerful about showing someone that you believe in them—even if they don't see it themselves. I let all of my clients "borrow my belief" in them and consistently highlight their wins and potential until they start to see themselves in the same positive light, get their confidence back, and begin to believe that their success is inevitable, no matter how long it takes.

My client Wendy referred her friend Melissa, and in my first conversation with her, she mentioned that one of the things she loved about Wendy was the fact that she *always* called Melissa out when she was speaking negatively about herself or selling herself short. If you don't yet have a Wendy in your life, start to *be* her to your friends and foster that kind of support in your own friend group.

Having a board of advisors: a mentor(s) and/or trusted professional(s) and a community of like-minded friends who, together, provide guidance, accountability, and support will help you become—and stay—committed, confident, and consistent in pursuit of your weight-loss goals and lifestyle that will make the changes stick.

Getting support does *not have* to mean spending money. Doing so may make sense for you and improve your experience and the quality of your results, but if you've already honed the skill of taking compassionate ownership of your life (more on that in the next chapter); you're ready, willing, and able to take action on free advice from trusted professionals (like in this book!); and you have a strong peer support system around you, you can absolutely be successful without spending another dime.

As I mentioned earlier, most women *don't* have great support systems, *aren't* in the habit of following through on their self-boundaries or taking compassionate ownership of their results, and tend to struggle without some amount of external accountability and guidance. Even if those don't sound like they apply to you, there may still be room for improvement if you want to take things from good to great.

If that does sound like you, don't use it against yourself. Asking for help doesn't mean you can't reach your goals on your own; it means you see the value in getting there easier, faster, and with more fun along the way.

I've mentioned that when I decided to write this book, I immediately sought out the comprehensive support I knew would benefit me to make it the best book possible. I had the confidence to believe I *could* do it on my own, but also the experience and humility to know that having a board of advisors would help: experienced and qualified professionals, external accountability, and a community of peers to learn from, teach, and with whom to connect.

Without a doubt, this book is better, and the writing process was more enjoyable, because I chose to ask for help and surround myself with comprehensive support.

Professionals

The first person you need on your advisory board is a trusted professional who can help you put together a road map to follow that is unique to YOU.

Think of the GPS in your car. It offers you different routes and information about why you may want/not want to take them. When you inevitably do make a wrong turn, it helps you reroute and course correct so you don't spiral off a cliff or turn back around to go home.

Your GPS doesn't do the driving *for* you, but it helps immensely with getting to your destination in a timely fashion and with as few frustrations and detours as possible.

It's appealing to want someone or something to do the work for you, but YOU need to be the one in the driver's seat, calling the shots and making decisions, and learning new skills.

So what *kind* of professional support do you need? I don't know you as a unique individual to answer that, but I will share with you some options so you can see what stands out. (Just like you probably have a preferred deli slicer and "hair gal," it may take a little bit of trial and error to find your person/people, but it'll be well worth it when you do.)

If your biggest struggle is knowing what to eat, specifically for a medical condition, consider working with a **Registered Dietitian (RD)**. You can likely get a referral through your insurance, and they're the only nutrition professionals qualified to treat medical conditions.

If your biggest struggle is knowing what to do in the gym, an in-person or virtual **Personal Trainer** may be the best bet. This person can write an exercise program for you, help ensure you're moving with safe and effective form, using heavy enough weights, and adjust the program to maximize results as you go.

If your whole life feels kind of like a dumpster fire, and you know it's going to be really hard to make headway with the exercise and nutrition "Big Rocks" until you address some other areas of your life (relationships, job, getting in your own way), then a **Life** or **Mindset Coach** may be a good fit.

If you're struggling with past traumas and need help introspecting and analyzing them in an effort to resolve and move past them, a **Therapist** or **Psychologist** may be a good fit.

If you know (or suspect) you have an eating disorder, someone who can guide you through the treatment and recovery process may be/include an **RD, therapist, or more.**

My Gone For Good program combines access to a Registered Dietitian, Exercise Physiologist, Personal Trainers, Life & Mindset Coaches, and Nutrition & Accountability coaches. Outside of individuals with specific medical conditions or those who would benefit from therapy first (or in conjunction), an option like what my business, EA Coaching, provides is the most comprehensive support available.

Like-Minded Peers

The next person or people you need on your advisory board are like-minded individuals who have similar goals and enough in common with you to be able to relate to your challenges and help support you through them. You don't want a group of women who are *exactly* like you because different personalities, experiences, and skill sets provide you alternative perspectives. Having women who can lift you up when you're down, celebrate your wins with you, and for whom you do the same will drastically improve your consistency, commitment, and confidence.

Prior to adding a group component to my coaching, I would spend hours on one-on-one calls with clients, many of whom would be facing the same challenges but would tell me, "I just feel like I'm the only person who . . ."

It's so important that you have an outlet where you feel comfortable being open, honest, and vulnerable with other women who get it and can help you see that you're *not* alone.

Not only do peers help normalize the changes you're making that might seem really "weird" to your current friends, but they also help normalize the ups and downs that are par for the course but are hard to find on social media where everyone is only sharing the ups!

Another benefit of peer support (and access to a *team* of coaches) is having the opportunity to learn the same things in different ways. Sometimes when you hear a message directed at someone else or phrased differently, you're more open to applying it than if it were coming from your own coach. For instance, hearing what's worked for another mom, whether she has a similar or completely different job or family dynamic, can help you apply the ideas and principles to your own life.

One of the things I enjoy the most about our client community is watching more seasoned clients step into this advisory role with newer clients. Not only is it comforting for newer clients to have a "big sister" type relationship with someone whose success they can see and aspire to, it helps the more seasoned client see how much she's learned and how far she's come, even if she's not yet where she wants to be.

How do you find people for your advisory board?

You can press the "easy" button and join a program like Gone For Good, where it's all included for you.

Or you can piecemeal one together from here and there, which is likely to be a lengthier process but can be just as effective.

I'd start by securing your trusted professional, as he or she may have an aspect of community involved in his or her services (for example, if you get a trainer at a gym, it's easy to tap in to the network of peers who also work with your trainer or suggest a small group of similarly minded peers).

Depending on where you live, it may be easy to find like-minded women local to you or it may make more sense to create more virtual connections. (When I originally wrote this chapter, I was living in northern Germany and did not speak German, so the bulk of my support was online. Now I'm living in San Diego where I know I'll form many in-person relationships).

It's okay for your wants, needs, and people on your advisory board to change with time and as *you* change. Keep in mind that connection and support is something we **all** need, *forever*.

While you don't always need to have professional guidance or community support, there are always benefits to having a team in your corner—humans are social beings!

My client Jonna is the perfect example of this. Her advisory board has changed numerous times over the last few years: she lost her first 20 pounds with a local nutritionist, spent over a year in our community during COVID, and now has a strong in-person gym community that's exactly what she needs for where she is now.

Your advisory board doesn't have to look a certain way; don't judge yourself for however it shapes up. You may have some people who are near you and some whom you never meet in person; if they're the people you need, they're the people you need. Give yourself the opportunity to get your needs met, however that looks right now.

Just like you need to make a lifelong commitment to your health, support will always be a part of that.

Although it's your responsibility to get yourself to your goals (more on that in the next chapter), that doesn't mean you have to do it alone.

Journal Prompts

It's time to think about and put together your own advisory board:

What do you need from your friends, family, and coworkers?

What professional help do you need?

Do you have an existing peer group, or do you need one?

Where can you find those people?

Action Steps

Reach out.

Communicate your needs.

Find people who will make losing weight and keeping it off easier, faster, and more fun along the way.

CHAPTER 10

COMPASSIONATE OWNERSHIP

"It was just another hard week," Dana sighed. From the minute she picked up the phone, I could tell she was upset. It's common, and totally normal, for clients to get frustrated by obstacles, especially early on in coaching.

While Dana was facing her fair share of them, they were nothing out of the ordinary, and dwelling on how hard they made things for her wasn't productive or fun.

Coaching is largely about listening, asking questions, and helping the client make their own decisions, so that's what I did.

"Tell me more," I encouraged her.

"Well, for starters, I know I've told you before that my husband does all our cooking. He just does *not* want to change how we eat. What am I supposed to do? Not eat what he makes?"

She went on, "And now that the weather is getting nicer, we're out on the boat every weekend and socializing with our neighbors. Including my one neighbor who's this Skinny Minny that wears these tiny jean shorts with her bikini top and I know all the husbands can't help but stare at her."

"I remember you mentioning her."

"She doesn't need to worry about what she eats or how much she drinks. It's not fair!"

These challenges, and others like them, were recurring topics of conversation over the course of our six months together and, over time, Dana was able to overcome all of them.

The first thing we had to do, though, was help her develop the foundational skill of compassionate ownership. This is what would allow her to say, "It's okay that I'm having a hard time and don't know the answer to this yet. I can and will figure out what to do."

Developing compassionate ownership would mean Dana would stop being so hard on herself for being less than perfect and not having all the answers, while also taking responsibility for learning the new skills and tools that would help her overcome her challenges, grow as a person, and make the changes necessary to create the results she wanted.

She needed to not be so hard on herself for where she was now. The decisions she'd made in the past were ones that *did* once serve her, even if they no longer were.

She needed to not beat herself up because she wasn't the family chef or because her husband was resistant to changing her diet.

She needed to not compare herself to her neighbor or make her neighbor's existence mean she couldn't *also* be fit and healthy.

Instead, she needed to learn how to change from a place of love, acceptance, and acknowledgement that she was worthy and deserving of more than the life she was currently living, not from a place of resentment, shame, or comparison.

She needed to learn how to take back control of her life.

She needed to understand that while her current circumstances weren't necessarily her fault, it was her *responsibility* to learn how to change the things about herself and her life with which she wasn't happy.

She needed to recognize that no one could do the work for her, and while nothing was going to magically change overnight to make her challenges disappear, she *did* have control over more than she thought.

She needed to have ownership of her actions, attitude, and effort.

One of the first agreements we made was that she wouldn't get down on herself or wallow in her excuses and would only use the past to help her learn, grow, and move forward toward her goals. She recognized that what she had done before—a combination of expecting perfection and being too hard on herself while also making lots of excuses for why she couldn't change—hadn't worked. She needed the inverse of all of that. To take responsibility for reaching her goals while also treating herself with the same kindness and understanding she'd extend to any other person.

This is compassionate ownership.

Compassionate ownership helps you develop consistency, commitment, and confidence. It helps you learn and master the "Big Rocks." It helps you create and lean on your support system. It helps with *everything* we've covered so far, as well as the skills and tools we'll cover in the rest of the book.

You might be thinking that you already give yourself way *too much* grace and let yourself off the hook too often. That you need someone to be hard on you because the only thing that will help you overcome your "natural laziness" and "lack of discipline" is a drill sergeant to berate you into submission.

But it's not.

Not consistently doing the "Big Rocks" or upholding your personal boundaries are signs you're not taking ownership, not that you're lazy, lacking discipline, or that you don't deserve compassion.

Many weight-loss programs focus on taking extreme ownership in a hardcore and cut-and-dried way that exacerbates the existing all-or-nothing thinking most women already experience. They end up feeling ashamed for falling slightly short of perfection or being unwilling to sacrifice everything else in their lives to reach their weight-loss goals.

On the other end of the spectrum, you have those preaching that you should never want to lose weight and should only ever lean into your intuition and eat whatever you want. This can make you feel guilty for wanting to change and be so woo-woo or touchy-feely that you never feel empowered to take action toward your weight-loss goal.

What you actually need to lose weight in a healthy and sustainable way—and for good—is to learn how to live in the middle of the spectrum that has these extremes at either end. Compassionate ownership is what exists in the middle. Sometimes you need more of one than the other, but you always need a combination of the two.

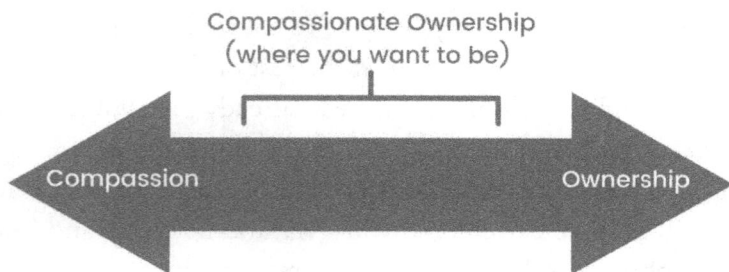

Compassionate Ownership
(where you want to be)

Compassion

Ownership

Building the skill of compassionate ownership first will help you see that any challenge you're facing has solutions that you are capable of figuring out and implementing. As you start to see your obstacles in this new way, you're one step closer to the tools and skills that will help.

We'll dive more into the other skills and tools in Part 3, but for the time being, what I want you to know is that compassionate ownership allows you to:

- Develop the self-awareness to pinpoint exactly what obstacles are holding you back from lasting results.

- Foster a growth mindset, which means believing that solutions to your challenges exist and you can learn new things and get better at them with time, effort, and persistence. You embrace and learn from challenges, stay committed through obstacles, and are inspired, rather than threatened, by other people's success.

- Develop your own Obstacle Toolbox: a mental "container" that holds all of the skills and tools you currently possess or acquire in the future that will help you lose weight, keep it off, and overcome future challenges.

- Become someone who's not easily derailed by life's challenges, isn't all-or-nothing, and who exhibits the consistency, commitment, and confidence to get results that last a lifetime.

- Develop the unshakeable confidence that you can and will reach your weight-loss—and any other—goal, no matter what life throws your way.

Even though it might not feel natural yet, start trying on the identity of someone who accepts that she is human and doesn't know everything but still believes she can learn new things, figure stuff out, and doesn't need to accept the status quo of her life.

"To know and not do, is not to know."
—Johann Wolfgang von Goethe

Identifying Your Values

Taking compassionate ownership and having a growth mindset to build the skills and tools to fill up your personal Obstacle Toolbox are lifelong pursuits.

It takes ongoing maintenance to keep up with anything that's important to you, from relationships, to a garden, to your home, even if you know those things can be replaced or rebuilt. Our vehicles are better off with routine maintenance like oil changes and tire rotations, but worst case, we run our cars into the ground and eventually need a new one. It's much cheaper, easier, and better to take care of the house you already own, but if you don't, well, you can always move! Relationships? Of course it's nice to have long-lasting ones that you nurture for decades . . . but if you don't want to put in the work to do that, you can always start swiping on your phone to find a new one.

Your body is the only thing that you are guaranteed to have your entire life, and that *can't* be replaced (at least not completely or easily), making taking care of yourself and your health the most important kind of maintenance there is.

If you feel like there's a disconnect between what you *say* you value and what your actions would lead someone to believe, using your values, vision for the future, and "Why" from Chapter 5 as filters for making decisions will help you show up as the person you want to be.

Regardless of whether you want to lose or maintain your weight, you need to be someone for whom health ranks among your top handful of values. Don't worry if you don't currently feel like or identify as a health-minded person. It's as easy as just deciding that's who you are and starting to act accordingly. Everything we've covered so far and in the rest of this book will help you do just that.

"Happiness is when what you think, what you say, and what you do are in harmony."
—Mahatma Gandhi

As I've mentioned, during my freshman year of college at Boston University I gained almost 40 pounds. I loved swiping into the dining hall midway through lunch, sampling all the comfort foods I wasn't used to having such easy access to, and hanging out with my friends until the staff changed the buffet over to the dinner options and we could eat all over again—while only paying for one meal!

Between those regular indulgences and the habit of getting stoned and ordering late night pineapple and black olive pizza that helped me bond with my new roommate, the weight just piled on.

I didn't notice at first, but it wasn't long before my pants were snug and I snuck over to a thrift shop on Comm Ave to buy what I called "fat pants" so I didn't have to wear baggy sweats all the time.

Once again, it wasn't long before *those* got snug, and I found myself wearing nothing but elastic waistbands.

Going back home to Maine that summer, I remember telling myself, "I forgot who I was for a while" as I worked to get consistently active again (it was much easier without the dining hall and munchies!).

Having such a strong identity as a fit and healthy person was the key to getting back to the behaviors that helped me get the weight off.

Identifying as a healthy person doesn't mean living in all-or-nothing extremes where you're constantly stressing over the "right" decision; it means making choices aligned with your health goals (both mental and physical) *most* of the time. It means looking *forward* to getting back to consistently applying the "Big Rocks" in your life because you love how you look and feel when you do.

Don't worry if you don't feel like that person yet. Just by following the Gone For Good formula, taking compassionate ownership, and filling up your Obstacle Toolbox, you will become someone who values her health and acts accordingly, day in and day out, without it feeling forced.

One of the best ways to pinpoint the obstacles standing between you and weight loss that lasts is to first get clear on your core values and use them as a litmus test for determining where there's a disconnect between those and your actions.

The following exercise will help you identify your values and see how your day-to-day choices are a reflection of those values. The journaling prompts will help you start to self-identify current obstacles and how to overcome them with a variety of skills and tools.

Assignment

Go through the Core Values list below and circle the top five that feel really important and meaningful to you right now.

Accountability	Fun	Perseverance
Achievement	Generosity	Personal
Adaptability	Giving back	fulfillment
Adventure	Grace	Power
Altruism	Gratitude	Pride
Ambition	Growth	Recognition
Authenticity	Harmony	Reliability
Balance	Health	Resourcefulness
Beauty	Home	Respect
Being the best	Honesty	Responsibility
Belonging	Hope	Risk-taking
Career	Humility	Safety
Caring	Humor	Security
Collaboration	Inclusion	Self-discipline
Commitment	Independence	Self-expression
Community	Initiative	Self-respect
Compassion	Integrity	Serenity
Competence	Intuition	Service
Confidence	Job security	Simplicity
Connection	Joy	Spirituality
Contentment	Justice	Sportsmanship
Contribution	Kindness	Stewardship
Cooperation	Knowledge	Success
Courage	Leadership	Teamwork
Creativity	Learning	Thrift
Curiosity	Legacy	Time
Dignity	Leisure	Tradition
Diversity	Love	Travel
Environment	Loyalty	Trust
Efficiency	Making a	Truth
Equality	difference	Understanding
Ethics	Nature	Uniqueness
Excellence	Openness	Usefulness
Fairness	Optimism	Vision
Faith	Order	Vulnerability
Family	Parenting	Wealth
Financial stability	Patience	Well-being
Forgiveness	Patriotism	Wisdom
Freedom	Peace	Write your own:
Friendship		

My top 5 core values right now are:

1. _____

2. _____

3. _____

4. _____

5. _____

Journal Prompts

Is health on this list? Why or why not?

If it's not, what needs to be different so that it cracks the top five?

If it is, write for ten minutes about why it is important to you (if you have time, feel free to do this for all your top values).

Obstacle Toolbox

I use the term Obstacle Toolbox to refer to all the skills and tools you have or will hone in the future that directly impact weight loss and leading a healthy lifestyle, or that will help you more generally with consistency, commitment, and confidence as they relate to *any* goal you want to accomplish.

After reading Chapters 7 and 8, you know *what* to do, so the challenge is understanding what's preventing you from *doing* the "Big Rocks" with the consistency and commitment you need to reach your goal and the confidence to know you'll be able to stay there.

Learning to take compassionate ownership means peeling back the layers and addressing the root issues that are preventing you from doing the day-to-day habits that get results or from *continuing* to do those things, even after you've reached your goal!

The process of doing this may cause you to uncover beliefs about yourself and the world, past traumas, issues with your relationship, career, alcohol, and more that you might not like or have ever realized before.

Taking compassionate ownership means being willing to go where the process takes you even when those places are unexpected or don't initially seem related to losing weight but will make sense eventually.

For Dana, like for most clients, this led to some enlightening realizations. Take one conversation in which we explored her struggles with being consistent with her workouts and she realized the following:

"Has there ever been a time that you've enjoyed exercising?" I asked her.

"No. As a kid I was always teased in gym class for being uncoordinated and dreaded the times when we had to pick teams because I was always picked last."

"How do you think those experiences might be affecting your relationship with exercise now?"

"I guess I associate all exercise with that negativity. As an adult I've just always avoided anything that brought back those memories."

With this awareness, Dana and I were able to work on developing several skills and tools to help her improve her relationship with exercise and start being more consistent with her workouts. She learned how to show herself that she is safe and not at risk of being teased like she was as a child. She learned how to let go of the "exercise = harmful" belief that had served to protect her in the past but was now holding her back. She learned how to tune in to the ways that working out makes her feel *good* and to create new, positive associations with exercise. Once Dana became aware of just how much her past was affecting her present and future, it was easier for her to work through limiting beliefs in other areas of her life.

In this instance, compassionate ownership looked like being gentle with herself while exploring these painful childhood memories and also recognizing that it was up to her to no longer be held back by them and be willing to do the work to overcome them. Although this trip down memory lane wasn't directly related to weight loss, learning these skills and tools helped her be more consistent with the exercise "Big Rocks," which *did* contribute to losing weight, being healthier, and having more confidence.

Dana graduated from coaching after six months, and she's continued to hone the skill of compassionate ownership on her own. She now has the calm confidence of a woman who understands and accepts that her life is always in flux and that there are limits to what she can control and *also* knows that no matter what happens, she will be okay and is capable of using her Obstacle Toolbox to figure things out. That is what the skill of compassionate ownership will help you create as well.

Like many women, Dana's weight has fluctuated over the years. Weight gain is an area where many women are particularly hard on themselves. Dana now understands that weight fluctuations are normal and not the end of the world—and that she has the power to course correct at any time.

She knows that sometimes life feels hard, or she finds herself spread really thin and that it's unrealistic to think that she'll go through life without her weight/body ever changing, especially when she lets her "Big Rock" habits slip or defaults back into comforting behaviors that aren't focused on health, weight loss, or maintenance. Even though she knows the Gone For Good formula and has the tools and skills she needs, she *still* has times where her health ends up further on the back burner than she'd like it, and the scale reflects that.

Instead of beating herself up and running to the next fad diet, as she has done in the past, Dana is able to treat herself with compassion, take a deep breath, and remind herself, "It's okay." She takes ownership by noticing what's going on, reminding herself that with her Obstacle Toolbox, she's equipped to handle all of life's challenges, and instead of panicking, just gets back to the "Big Rock" habits that always help her get to where she wants to be.

Skills & Tools

Since Part 3 of this book is all about helping you develop the skills and tools that will help you lose weight for good, what I want you to consider for right now is that you likely have gaps in your skillset that you need to address in order to overcome the weight loss challenges you're facing now and will in the future.

I don't mean gaps in the sense that you're not sure what to eat or do for workouts, but the skills that will help you *do* those things consistently, like setting and upholding boundaries, practicing better time management, planning ahead, or learning how to stop comparing your journey to other people's. I know these might not sound like the issues you normally associate with trying to lose weight, but the "beneath the surface" challenges are what are *actually* preventing weight loss that lasts, and developing the necessary skills will help you lose weight and keep it off.

> *"Knowing is not enough; we must apply.*
> *Willing is not enough; we must do."*
> —*Johann Wolfgang von Goethe*

As such, any obstacle standing in your way is really just an opportunity to develop or hone new skills or practice applying new tools.

In this way, slip ups are a *good* thing because they allow you to identify the gaps and become smarter, more resilient, and better equipped to navigate similar (and inevitable) challenges in the future.

Tools are devices or implements used to carry out a particular function, like food-tracking apps and activity trackers.

Skills are the ability to use one's knowledge effectively and readily in execution or performance, like knowing how to cook and modify workouts around limitations.

Having both skills *and* tools means you're filling up your Obstacle Toolbox and are able to do a certain thing effectively, in order to accomplish something specific.

You already have many of the tools and skills you need (like organization or communicating your needs); you just may not be in the habit of recognizing your strengths or applying them to your health goals. For example, my client

Emily prided herself on being super organized at work but felt like a total disaster when it came to planning out the rest of her life. She felt like her work and home identities were completely separate, but once she realized she could apply her organizational skills to her exercise and nutrition habits and utilize tools like her Google calendar and iPhone reminders, her consistency and confidence went through the roof.

Compassionate ownership helps you recognize that you already possess or can learn the tools and skills you need to adjust accordingly as your life, circumstances, priorities, and goals change. Rather than grasping to a sinking ship because the "old" way is the only way you know, you recognize that you have the power to create new strategies, routines, or habits to achieve your goals. Compassionate ownership makes it a lot less stressful and overwhelming to troubleshoot the inevitable challenges you'll experience over the course of a lifetime.

Here's an example: just about everyone would benefit from learning and mastering the exercise and nutrition "Big Rocks." Exactly what that looks like, and the skills and tools one needs, may vary drastically from person to person and even within the same person at different seasons of her life!

Kate was a 30-something who was newly postpartum with her second baby in two years. She got in her daily steps while pushing her kids in the double stroller. She was grateful for at-home workout programs to take the thought out of strength training and, as needed, would substitute a cranky baby for a pair of dumbbells. Prioritizing protein and fiber while getting in enough calories to maintain her supply of breast milk meant using a meal-prep service for dinners and drinking a lot of smoothies she could sip on between *Cocomelon* and diaper changes.

Maria, on the other hand, was retired after 30 years as a postal worker. She had plenty of time on her hands and came to realize how much the structure of her work schedule had helped her get things done. To make sure she was getting her steps in, she formed a group of friends from church for walks three mornings per week. She was new to strength training, so she signed up for personal training at the community center to help her learn how to do so safely. Learning how to cook was a hobby she'd taken up with her husband in retirement, and she loved finding new recipes that they both enjoyed, knew were nutritious, and helped them hit their nutrition "Big Rocks."

Both women, like almost all of my clients, were strength training, walking, recovering, prioritizing protein and fiber, and eating the right number of calories for their needs. But what that looked like was very different for each of them, and both utilized a variety of skills and tools in order to be consistent with them.

Identifying Needs & Filling In Skill Gaps

How do you know where the gaps in your skillset are? How do you actually go about developing the tools you need to fill them in?

It starts with awareness of what you're currently doing and whether or not those actions support your core values and, specifically, your weight-loss goals.

Developing awareness requires you to be curious, collect data (as discussed in Chapter 8), reflect on it, and start identifying the opportunities you have to develop new skills and tools, or start applying ones you already have to a new situation.

Keeping a behavior awareness journal can help you pick up on patterns of behavior, like when you're most prone to giving in to temptation, emotional eating, or other self-sabotaging behaviors.

Learning to delay gratification is another important piece of taking compassionate ownership. There are going to be times when what you want right *now* is at odds with your weight-loss goal and the future you want for yourself.

While you don't need to make long-term goal focused choices *all* the time, you do need to make them *most* of the time (remember the 85% sweet spot from Chapter 4)—if you want to reach your goal, anyway. Learning how to pause in the moment and ask yourself what you *really* want, and which choice best supports that goal, is just one more tool to add to your Obstacle Toolbox.

Once you're aware of your patterns and triggers, you're one step closer to breaking those cycles and choosing different outcomes. You may notice that you go through a period of having awareness but not yet having the skills or tools to overcome them, which can be incredibly frustrating.

As you begin practicing different coping skills and strategies for breaking the loop, remember that it takes trial and error, a willingness to experiment, some reflection on what's working or not, and persistence in continuing to practice, tweak, and refine over and over again, remembering to be both compassionate *and* to take ownership along the way. As you do, you'll be more and more confident in your abilities to most consistently make different choices that result in better outcomes and help you lose weight, keep it off, and pursue other goals.

Journal Prompts

Brain dump all the excuses you make or situations you have let derail you in the past.

Brainstorm solutions for everything on that list.

What will help you overcome those or similar obstacles in the future?

What do you need to do/learn/have in order to implement those solutions?

What skills, tools, or people would help you?

Using Skills & Tools When You Need Them (And Stopping When You Don't)

Understanding that you only need to use tools when they serve a purpose helps erase the overwhelm of starting.

Wouldn't it be much easier to consistently track your food if you knew it wasn't a lifelong commitment but a tool for developing awareness that you would use for a few months to help you reach your weight-loss goal in a way you could then maintain without tracking?

Wouldn't it be easier to rid your kitchen of temptations if you knew it didn't mean you could never have snacks or treats again, and that shaping your environment was simply a tool to help you break some old habits that were making it harder to lose weight?

Being a military family, we move every few years, which means having to hang our artwork all over again with each new home. Imagine for a minute that my husband Grey and I have stopped bickering about placement for long enough to actually get a good system down with the hammer and the nails and we've successfully finished half the house.

Would it make sense for us to decide to stop using the hammer and see what other kind of blunt object we could use to whack in the nails? Not really, right? Why wouldn't we just keep using the tools and the system that's working—until the job is done?

It's important not to stop using a tool before you're ready. Many women struggle with the transition out of food tracking because they convince themselves that, by now, they *should* have learned enough to be successful without it. While that may be the case and there's no harm in experimenting (you can always pick a tool back up again), there's also no reason to rush yourself to be "done" with it when a particular tool is helping you feel good, be successful, and see results without feeling deprived. There's just no point after which you're beyond or too advanced for a given tool.

Recap

Remember that compassionate ownership is a skill you can practice *any* time and that filling your Toolbox with skills and tools and knowing when to use them and put them back is an ongoing process. Give yourself grace, be willing to be a beginner, learn from your "failures," and prepare to be blown away by your physical and mental progress when you look back and see how far you've come.

The upcoming chapters are devoted to helping you fill up your Obstacle Toolbox with skills and tools and start implementing the Gone For Good formula in your life.

PART 3

By now, you know that consistency, commitment, and confidence are the 3 Cs of success. You understand that walking, strength training, rest, calories, protein, and fiber are the exercise and nutrition "Big Rocks." You recognize the benefits of having comprehensive support and how taking compassionate ownership can help you develop those attributes. It's time to start developing the skills and tools that will help you implement the Gone For Good formula in a way that's specific to YOU.

The first skill we'll develop is learning how to set better goals.

CHAPTER 11

GOAL SETTING

"What New Year's Resolutions are you setting?" read the early December post in a popular Facebook group for moms.

Attached was a picture of a handwritten list on one of those grocery list pads that sticks to your fridge so you can jot down when you run out of milk. The original poster had three goals written down on this list: drink less, be more present, lose weight.

She'd also written the numbers 4 and 5, but those lines were blank, which was why she was turning to her 37,000 closest friends. She hoped some of the other ladies would share goals she could add to her list.

Hundreds of women responded. They, too, wanted to drink less, be more present, and lose weight. They also wanted to exercise more, get organized, be craftier, start playing tennis, spend less money, travel more, find new jobs, and have more fun.

It was hard not to be inspired by the positive changes so many women were committed to making (once the new year rolled around).

I couldn't help but wonder, though, how many of them would follow through and start—and how many of those would be consistent for long enough to actually accomplish them.

Most people make a handful of common mistakes when setting goals that reduce the likelihood they'll actually follow through and accomplish them. Fortunately, they're easy to avoid and by the end of this chapter, you'll know how to do just that and set specific, realistic, goals that set you up for success.

Goal-Setting Problem #1: Setting Goals You Don't Actually Care About

My first job after college was working in a commercial gym as a personal trainer. A lot of us were pretty inexperienced, so we did a lot of mock consults with one another to practice selling our personal training packages.

Whenever I was the pretend client, I said my goal was to lose five pounds and build muscle. Neither of those things were particularly important to me at the time (though building muscle should have been!); I said they were my goals because it felt like what I was *supposed* to say.

Whether you feel societal, familial, social, or personal pressure to look—or be—a certain way, a certain weight, or a certain size, you do not need to give into it. Consider this your official permission to no longer set goals because you feel like you should, rather than because they're things you actually care about.

So if weight loss isn't something you really want, then guess what? YOU DON'T NEED TO HAVE A WEIGHT-LOSS GOAL.

There is so much more to you, to your life, to your worth, than the number on a scale. If setting a weight-loss goal feels like a distraction from things you *actually* care about, you don't have to have one.

Setting goals that aren't meaningful to you makes it a struggle to be committed and make a consistent effort to achieve them, leaving you frustrated and disappointed.

If setting a weight-loss goal feels like the first step down the path of creating the identity and confidence of the person you want to be, by all means, set one.

Outside of the scale, other health-related goals may include:

- losing inches
- fitting into your clothes
- having more energy
- being stronger
- having better endurance
- being more consistent
- rebuilding your reputation with yourself
- having more confidence
- having an identity shift
- having better health markers
- being happier and in better moods more often
- being an inspiration to others
- knowing your success here and at any goal is inevitable
- pursuing your dreams/passions
- not picking yourself apart in the mirror
- having better self-talk
- setting a healthier example for your kids
- being less preoccupied with your body

- having more bandwidth to devote to other areas of your life that are more enjoyable

Solution: Identify Goals You *Do* Care About

Whatever your goal is, you want it to be something you feel deeply connected to. Understanding your "Why," the emotional reason that your goal is important to you, is crucial for staying committed to it.

Why do you need to reach your goal no matter how long it takes or how hard it feels sometimes? How will your life change for the better as a result? You may have already dug into this when we talked about it in Chapter 5, but if not, now is the time.

Here are some reasons my clients have shared:

1. HEALTH & LONGEVITY RELATED

- I don't want to be on medication like my parents were.
- I don't want to die from a heart attack.
- I want to do what I can to make sure I live a long time so I can be around for my kids.
- I want to get back to the version of me that doesn't hurt all the time.

2. FAMILY RELATED

- I don't want to say in front of my kids what my mom said to me.
- I want to be a role model for my kids and show them what a healthy, active lifestyle looks like.
- I want to be able to get on the floor and play with my grandkids.

3. **ENERGY, CONFIDENCE, and SUCCESS RELATED**

- I would like to feel better, have more energy, and get my confidence back.

- I don't want to feel self-conscious about my body in social settings.

- I want the confidence that I know will make me more successful in all aspects of my life.

4. **QUALITY OF LIFE and IMPACT RELATED**

- I want to have the bandwidth to serve my community, something I don't have right now because I'm constantly thinking about my health; I believe I'm a better role model when I'm healthier.

- I want to not be obsessed with my weight so that I can concentrate on fulfilling my purpose in life.

Journaling Prompts

What is your goal?

What does your goal represent to you?

How is it about so much more than the goal itself?

What is your driving force, and how can you keep that at top of mind when your initial motivation and enthusiasm are waning?

If you didn't already do the 5 Whys exercise in Chapter 5, do it now:

Write your goal and then ask the first "why" (Why do I want to _____?)

Whatever the answer is, you then ask "why" to that answer. Repeat the process five times.

Each time you do, like peeling back the layers of an onion, you'll be getting closer to the root reason that the goal is important to you.

What is your Why?

Goal-Setting Problem #2: Being Too Vague & Focusing Solely On Outcomes

The goals everyone was sharing in that Facebook post sounded great! Who wouldn't want to learn a new language, be healthier, and have more money?

The problems here are two-fold:

1. Vague goals leave you unclear on the *outcome* you're after—what reaching the goal actually looks like.
2. Vague outcomes leave you unclear on the *behaviors* that will help you reach the goal—what day-to-day actions will lead to your desired result.

Without being specific about what you want, how will you know what to do to get there or when you have?

When you think about being a Healthy Person, what exactly is it that you're picturing? What does "be healthier" actually mean to you?

How will you know if you've been more present?

How much more money do you want to have saved and by when?

When you set a weight-loss goal, is seeing *that* specific number on the scale the win, in and of itself? Or do you want to fit into your favorite work pants, be able to comfortably zip up your ski jacket, or wear clothes that aren't in the plus-sized section?

When you say you want to be healthier, do you mean you want to get your blood pressure back into normal range? Get off a medication? Be able to run a mile without stopping or do five push-ups on your toes?

The more specific you can be with exactly the outcome you're after, the easier it'll be to focus on the actual behaviors that will help you reach it!

Solution: Be Specific With Outcomes And Focus on Behaviors

If you've done the writing exercises in Chapter 5 and the section above, you already have a lot more clarity on what's important to you and the specific results you desire. Understanding your weight-loss time frame as we covered in Chapter 4 will help you have realistic expectations for how long it will take you to reach your outcome goal. (If you haven't done these exercises yet, or need a refresher, do that now!)

Having a clear outcome goal is important because it serves as your compass. At any time, you can refer to that goal to gauge whether you are moving toward or away from it. You can use it to filter decisions and stay focused on what you want long term.

Once you know the outcome you're after, it's important to shift focus to behavior goals or the day-to-day actions that, when done consistently, will make reaching your outcome goal all but inevitable.

Goal-Setting Problem #3: Doing Too Much At Once

The New Year's Resolution post I mentioned at the beginning of the chapter, where hundreds of women shared their goals, took place in early December. It's easy to set goals when there's distance between stating them and putting in the work to achieve them.

The first issue is that this distance made it easy to set way more goals than would actually be possible to accomplish all at once. It's common to think that next year, next month, or next week you won't be so busy or spread so thin and will have more time to pursue your goals.

Odds are, though, that your life next year, next month, or next week is going to be pretty similar to your life now. You might have a lot of things you want to accomplish—and you *can*—but you need to be realistic about the bandwidth you have available. You can't pursue all of your goals all at once.

You're just not going to become fluent in Spanish while also heading the PTA, getting promoted at work, starting a side hustle, learning how to ice skate, and losing 50 pounds before your summer birthday like my client Bella tried to do. You have to prioritize and take a more gradual approach.

You will accomplish so much more by setting fewer goals each week, month, or quarter that you devote a good chunk of energy to and then either accomplish or make routine enough that you can stack another thing on top of it without feeling overwhelmed. If you keep trying to do everything at once, you risk getting overwhelmed, giving up, and finding yourself back in the all-or-nothing cycle.

Prior to working with me, Bella would write a whole laundry list of goals like the ones above that she wanted to accomplish by her next birthday, and she would go all-in on them right after the previous year's party. For the first month, she would be really focused on, well, everything. She would diligently do her Duolingo exercises, research business ideas during short breaks from her day job, wake up early to get her in her workouts, and stay up late making cookies for bake sales.

Paying more attention to her diet, getting outside, and moving more did help her feel better within a few weeks but the reality of spreading herself too thin, not sleeping enough, and having so much on her mind started to take its toll.

She was constantly tired from burning the candle at both ends. She felt like she was just going through the motions during her workouts, she wasn't actually retaining much from her Spanish lessons, she hadn't gotten past the research stage on any of her business ideas, and, on more than one occasion, she'd forgotten important ingredients in her baked goods and had to start all over.

Bella felt like she was doing a lot but none of it particularly well and like she didn't have enough time to really make a dent in *any* of her goals, let alone accomplish all of them at the same time. When she inevitably hit an obstacle like one of her kids getting sick, an unexpected work deadline, or her husband went on a work trip, things fell apart. Every year.

She was in the habit of going all-in on all her goals *and* all the behaviors that would help her reach them, all at once. This "jumping in" method was a drastic shift from what she'd been doing just weeks prior and was the exact reason she kept falling short of those goals and setting them again the following year.

By the time Bella reached out to me, she knew she couldn't keep doing the same thing and expecting a different outcome somehow, but doing less felt like she wasn't trying hard enough or couldn't possibly work.

Solution: Take a More Gradual Approach to Behavior Goals

Because she was coachable, Bella agreed to take a more gradual approach and prioritize the behavioral changes she wanted to make, adding them in one or two at a time in an order that made sense for her. Focusing on smaller behavior goals every two to four weeks like eating three servings of veggies per day, getting 8,000 steps, or carving out one to two hours per week to devote to business development, gave her the opportunity to make each behavior feel easier and more habitual before adding another.

Instead of fizzling out, her consistency, commitment, and confidence improved with each new habit she built. By the end of that year, Bella had lost 25 pounds and as many inches, was wearing a size eight, sleeping better, had more energy, and could carry on a basic conversation in Spanish. She decided that she actually *didn't* want a side business and instead wanted to devote that time and energy to being more present with her family and volunteering for (non-bake sale related) school events. She felt better and more accomplished than she had in years and knew that the progress she was making toward her outcome goals was sustainable because she had added the behaviors gradually, which allowed her to do them more consistently and with less effort.

Think about what you have the bandwidth for right now, in *real* life, not what would be nice if you didn't have a job and kids and responsibilities. Start there.

Since you're three-fourths of the way through this book, I'm going to assume your health or weight-loss goal is among your top priorities. Do you have other outcome goals you are willing to back burner for the time being so that you can give the necessary time and energy to your weight-loss goal? That's not to say that you need to pause all other goals, just that you'll be more successful in all areas if you don't take on too much at once and allow yourself to take a more gradual approach, both to the behaviors within a specific outcome *and* to the number of outcomes you're pursuing at the same time.

Journaling Prompts

What are ALL the outcome goals you'd like to accomplish in the next year, including but not limited to health/weight loss?

Which of these outcome goals are the most important to you and why? Which are you willing to deprioritize (*for now*) in order to pursue those?

When it comes to prioritizing the behaviors that will help you reach your weight-loss goal, the most important thing is that you just start. There is no perfect order of operations, and what makes the most sense for *you* will depend on variables like your personality, where you're starting, your goal, and more. The exact approach you take will be different from other people and that's okay; there are a variety of ways to reach the same destination.

You're familiar with the exercise and nutrition "Big Rocks" from Chapters 7 and 8, and I do recommend that those are where you focus your time and energy when it comes to weight loss, but if starting with even one of those feels like too big of a step from where you are now, that's fine!

For example, you may know that your nighttime snacking is the biggest contributor to your excess calories coming in and would rather address that before starting to tackle the nutrition "Big Rocks" of calories, protein, and fiber.

One useful exercise is to brain dump all the behavior goals you'd like to tackle, whether that's focusing on the "Big Rocks," breaking habits you know aren't serving you, or whatever else comes up for you that may or may not be directly related to weight loss but could make it easier (like prioritizing sleep).

From there, you can decide the approach you would like to take:

- **Top Down**—where you tackle the biggest challenges first, knowing that those will have the biggest impact on your weight loss, which will motivate you to keep going and likely make some of the smaller challenges obsolete.

- **Bottom Up**—where you start with smaller, easier changes to collect wins, build momentum, and help confidently tackle the bigger changes.

Keep in mind that your outcomes are a reflection of your efforts, so temper your expectations based on the size of the changes you're making. A gradual approach will lead to gradual weight loss that is more likely to last a lifetime. Being realistic with your expectations will help you stay consistent, committed, and confident that taking a gradual approach *will* help you reach your goal of losing weight and keeping it off.

Within the "Big Rocks," there are a variety of ways you can implement them:

- You may like the idea of having one exercise and one nutrition focus and gradually adding the other two of each as you feel ready. This could look like tracking your calories and hitting a daily step goal, and then adding a focus on protein and strength training once the first two feel easier.

- You may like the idea of starting with just exercise or just nutrition; for example, if you know you don't have much time or energy to devote to your weight-loss goal right now, so you choose to focus on hitting your calorie, protein, and fiber goals before carving out time for the exercise "Big Rocks."

- You may not be in the habit of doing any exercise, so you choose to create a consistent exercise routine first, knowing that doing so will make you more inclined to make better food choices and then you can focus on the nutrition "Big Rocks" from there.

There's no wrong way to approach your behavior goals, and it's more important *that* you take action rather than doing so in any specific way.

Journal Prompts

Brain dump your list of behavior goals.

Does a Top Down or Bottom Up approach appeal more to you? Why?

Which specific behavior goals will you start with? (If the "Big Rocks," which order will you go in? Will you focus on one exercise and one nutrition habit at the same time or work on one and then the other?)

Goal-Setting Problem #4: Repeating The All-or-Nothing Approach

Most of us default to what's familiar and "worked" before, whether that's a detox, WW, the 75 Hard challenge I used to help facilitate at the gym, or eliminating all processed foods. Generally, it's something drastic and restrictive that *does* help you lose some weight but also makes you very likely to put it right back on afterward.

Because most women don't have a plan to do things differently, they default to repeating what they've done before, which is typically an all-or-nothing approach that follows a pattern like this:

- **January**—Set weight-loss goal, commit to [insert diet here], lose weight, feel good
- **Feb/Mar**—Get burned out, have trouble sticking to [insert diet here], gain weight, feel bad

- **Apr/May**—Start thinking about summer, commit to [insert diet here], lose weight, feel good
- **Summer**—Don't want to think about [insert diet here] anymore, drink, eat, & socialize more, gain weight, feel bad
- **Early fall**—Panic before the holidays, commit to [insert diet here], lose weight, feel good
- **Holidays**—Don't want to deny yourself over the holidays, take a break from [insert diet here] overindulge, gain weight, feel bad
- **January**—repeat

Effort that spikes and plummets based on the time of year, your motivation, and other responsibilities on your plate does not create meaningful results. Instead, the oscillations cause you to fluctuate between feeling all-consumed by losing weight and being consumed by guilt and shame that you're not making any effort at all.

While you don't want drastic fluctuations in your efforts or commitment to your weight-loss goal, it *is* important to understand that neither your efforts nor your results will ever be perfectly steady.

As I mentioned previously, every area of our lives is in flux. Sometimes our kids demand more of our time. Sometimes it's our marriage, work, or any of a number of other important aspects of happy and fulfilling lives. It's important to acknowledge and anticipate that your efforts will ebb and flow based on other "life stuff" and to match your expectations to what is realistic given the circumstances.

If your busy season at work coincides with a major home renovation while one of your children is falling behind at school and you're advocating on her behalf, you will have less time and energy to give to your weight-loss journey. That's fine.

Effort Level

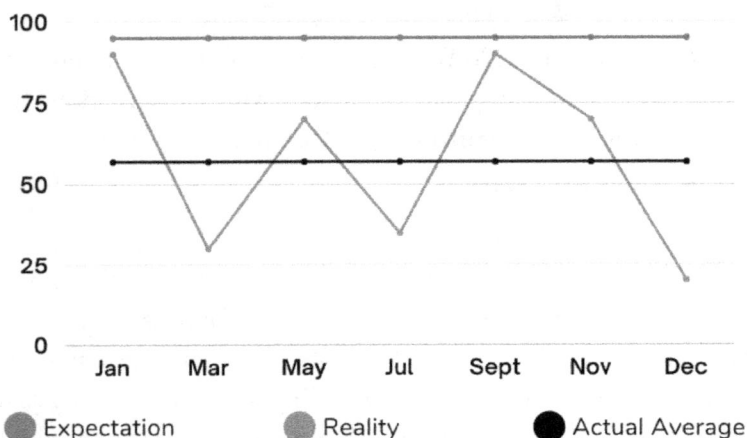

Expectation   Reality   Actual Average

Journal Prompts

What has been your weight-loss cycle in the past?

After how long do things start to fall apart and you lose focus? What has caused that to happen?

How does it feel when that happens?

How would you *like* losing weight to feel?

What thoughts or expectations do you need to reframe in order to commit to a gradual approach and gradual results?

Solution: Take a Surge-And-Cruise Approach

Since there will never be a time when you can focus solely on losing weight, you **must** learn to work *with* your life and continue to make your health a priority regardless of what's going on in the rest of your life.

This requires being:

- **Realistic**—taking into account all the other demands on your time & aspects of your life besides weight loss, not expecting yourself to give 100% all the time (aka living in the messy middle)
- **Flexible**—not following a ton of arbitrary "rules"
- **Focused on Sustainability**—not sacrificing your health or quality of life for the sake of seeing the scale move
- **Focused on Maintenance**—developing the mindset and lifestyle you need to make maintenance easy, while you're losing weight

Effort Level

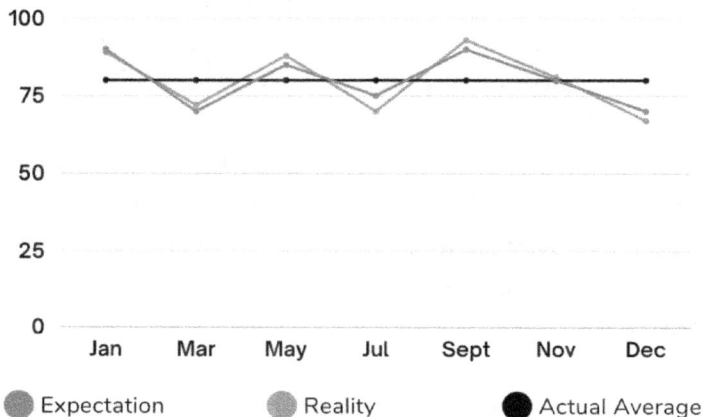

As we talked about in Chapter 3, overcoming your all-or-nothing mentality requires thinking about your efforts on a dial rather than an on-off switch. Sometimes you have to turn your dials up, and sometimes you have to turn them down. Rather than drastic swings in either direction, smaller adjustments will allow you to still average around the 85% threshold for seeing progress or maintaining the results you've already gotten.

Breaking your all-or-nothing mentality means not having to choose between being hyper-focused on weight loss or backsliding to where you started. It actually *is* possible to alternate between making progress and maintaining it.

My Surge & Cruise Method will help you do that.

Learning to Surge and Cruise allows you to adjust your efforts based on what else is going on in your life and nearly always hit the weekly behavior goals you set for yourself because they're realistic to begin with.

Surging and Cruising are not drastically different. You can think about them like being on a boat. When you're Surging, you open the engine up and speed faster toward your destination. When you're Cruising, your boat is still floating and pointed in the right direction, you've just slowed down, perhaps because of weather (necessity) or a desire to enjoy other aspects of being out on the water.

Either way, you'll be doing the "Big Rocks," and your actions will be similar, but your effort and expectations shift from being progress focused and at or over 85% consistency to being maintenance focused and a little below 85% consistency:

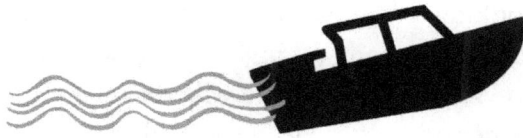

SURGE

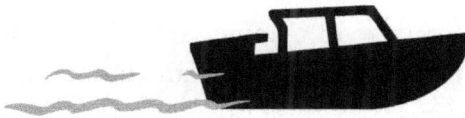

CRUISE

SURGING	CRUISING
Caloric Deficit—tracking your food accurately and consistently	Caloric Maintenance— maybe tracking, maybe not
Hitting protein goal Hitting fiber goal (ideally)	Prioritizing protein & fiber without necessarily tracking grams
8,000+ steps most days	As many steps as are feasible
3+ strength sessions/week	2+ strength sessions/week
1-3 rest days/week	1-3 rest days/week (or more!)
~½ body weight in ounces of water/day	~½ body weight in ounces of water/day
7+ hours of sleep	As much sleep as is feasible
Daily/weekly stress management/self-care	Daily/weekly stress management/self-care

Looking at the weeks, months, and year ahead can help you identify periods during which it will make more sense for you to Surge and when it will make more sense to Cruise. Cruise periods naturally give you "diet breaks" where you focus on maintaining where you are rather than losing, which help you build confidence that you will keep the weight off and stay committed and consistent during the surrounding Surge periods because you know those breaks are coming.

Although you can't predict what life is going to throw at you in the next couple of hours, let alone a year in advance, it's still useful to be proactive in mapping out your Surge and Cruise phases to the best of your ability at the moment.

Here's what a Surge-and-Cruise calendar might look like from a yearlong perspective:

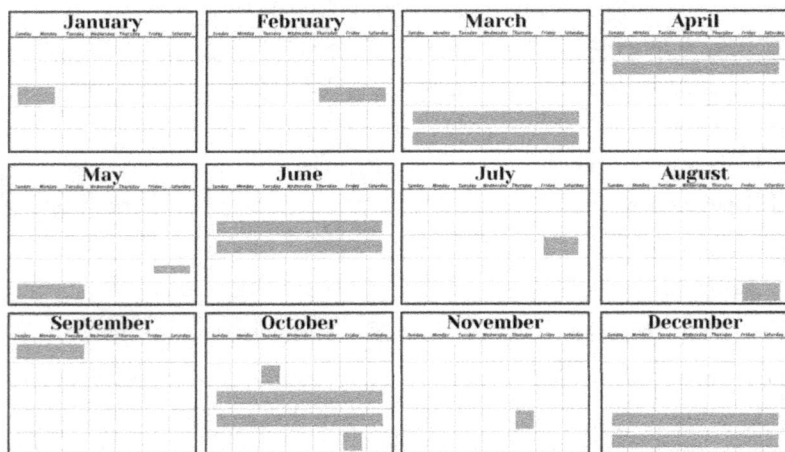

The blocked off dates are Cruise periods where you already know it would be difficult to Surge, such as planned vacations, holidays, or busy times at work, but it's fine to build in Cruise periods just because you know you could use a break. Open areas are where Surging will likely be easier, though not all of the remaining dates *need* to be devoted to Surging.

Keep in mind that things will pop up with varying amounts of notice, and the unexpected occurrences help you develop the skills of being able to think on your feet and not getting bent out of shape when things don't go according to plan. Creating a Surge-and-Cruise calendar is not set in –stone, and in fact, it's something you can update when you do your Life Admin, which we'll talk about in Chapter 12.

Creating Your Surge-and-Cruise Calendar

List out what you already know about your year, including vacations, work trips, busy seasons at work, holidays and special occasions, periods of change or transition, spouse travel, visitors, school breaks, etc.

Based on this, when does it make sense for you to Surge? When does it make sense for you to Cruise?

I understand this has been a doozy of a chapter and you may be feeling overwhelmed about setting the right outcome goals, prioritizing the right behaviors, and bringing it all together to create the lasting weight loss you're after. Don't worry! Coming up, we'll talk about creating the habit of "life admin" that you'll use to check in with yourself, make sure you're making progress toward your goals, tweak your outcome and behavior goals, and update your weekly, monthly, and annual plans.

CHAPTER 12

LIFE ADMIN

Lou has had an incredibly stressful and demanding job in education for the last seven years. She also has a 14-year-old son, 12-year-old daughter, and husband with his own demanding career. On top of that, they live in the Midwest near both her parents and in-laws, who are needing more help around the house these days.

When her kids were little, it felt like she was in survival mode 100% of the time. She couldn't even begin to think about starting to exercise, and any food she managed to eat was usually her kids' leftovers as she was cleaning up.

Once they were older, she went back to work and her drive to excel in her career monopolized any down time she gained from their both being in school.

Her kids got involved with sports and after-school activities, and she climbed the corporate ladder at work, leaving her more and more strapped for time as the years went on. Each January, she went through the motions of making weight-loss resolutions, knowing full well she had no capacity to actually follow through. The exercise equipment and cookbooks she bought to try to motivate herself were just collecting dust and taking up space in the house that had grown too small for two almost-teenagers.

Next came a move to a nicer neighborhood with a bigger house and yard to maintain, new neighbors to keep up with, and more pressure to continue to perform at work so they could afford their new lifestyle.

She had never felt like the biggest person in the room or like people were staring at or judging her. Now, making the rounds to meet her new neighbors left her riddled with insecurity as she realized most of the other women in the cul-de-sac were size-zero, stay-at-home moms with whom she felt like she had nothing in common.

She felt like she hadn't come up for air in more than a decade, and now that her kids were older and she had a bit more time, she barely recognized herself. She was constantly exhausted, regularly snapped at her kids for the smallest infractions, and couldn't remember the last time she had sex with her husband. She had dark bags under her eyes, her once thick and shiny hair was brittle and thin, and she'd somehow gained 75 pounds since her youngest was born.

Lou knew something had to change, but she wasn't sure what, which is why she reached out to me.

Though the specifics of Lou's life may be unique to her, the situation she was in is one to which millions of moms around the country can relate. Life seems to be going by at a million miles an hour, and you're spread so thin that you can't imagine doing anything more than just hanging on for the ride.

Just winging it and hoping for the best wasn't working for her, it's not working for you, and it's going to continue to not work.

Lou and I worked together on carving out time for "life admin," which is intentional time set aside each year (covered in the previous chapter), quarter, month, week, and day to reflect, set goals, and create specific actionable plans to accomplish them. These shorter-term check-ins with yourself allow you to figure out how you're progressing, identify what's going well, pinpoint where you're struggling, and figure out how to continue moving forward.

These short meetings with herself were a game changer for Lou and came to be something she looked forward to each week, as I know they will be for you.

Before we go over the specifics of exactly how to conduct your "life admin," let's first go over the forms of data you may want to collect to help you gauge your progress.

Progress Updates

When talking about weight loss, most women have a tendency to focus on the scale and use that as the primary means of determining success. The scale can be one useful metric to track, but it's incredibly helpful to also keep an eye on a variety of others for a few reasons:

- To help you see and take pride in progress that's *not* reflected on it, like losing inches or your clothes fitting better

- To help keep the scale in perspective so you're not feeling like your success is solely riding on the number that day

- To remind you that seeing a smaller number isn't the only thing driving you to make your health a priority (review Chapters 5 and 11 to remind yourself of your Why)

If you choose to track your scale weight, consider what frequency will help you collect useful data without being excessive. Some of my clients have weighed daily and enjoyed learning about their body's day-to-day fluctuations and how different foods, stress levels, or phases of their cycles impact the scale. Others choose not to use the scale at all. If you're not sure how often you'd like to use the scale, I would recommend starting with three to four times per week. This will allow you to see fluctuations and look at weekly averages without feeling like your weight is always at top of mind.

Whether or not you're using the scale, I recommend taking full body photos in addition to circumference measurements to help you see a more complete picture of the body composition changes you're experiencing. (I know you may feel reluctant to take photos of yourself and you don't *have* to, but they'll likely be something you're glad to have to look back on and see how far you've come).When you're prioritizing the "Big Rocks" of strength training and prioritizing protein, it's not unusual to lose inches and see changes in how your clothing is fitting even if the scale isn't moving much.

Common measurement sites are your neck, shoulders, chest, upper arm, hips, waist, thigh, and calf. Photos can be taken by recording yourself standing facing, parallel to, and away from the camera, and then taking screenshots in each position. Your book portal (www.estheravant.com/book-portal-signup) has a guide for taking progress pics and circumference measurements.

Other metrics you may decide to track include mood, energy levels, sleep quality or time to fall asleep, workout performance (speed you're able to run, distance you can run without stopping, output on your Peloton, weights you're able to use in your strength workouts, etc.), blood pressure, and A1C, to name a few. Choose a handful of metrics that will help you get a feel for whether you're making progress in the ways that matter to you the most.

In addition to metrics like these, I recommend keeping a running list of Non-Scale Victories to help you see all your wins that aren't necessarily scale or aesthetic based. This can include literally anything you notice that indicates you are becoming healthier, happier, or more confident. Some of my favorites from clients have been:

- I was able to zip knee-high boots over my calves for the first time!
- I noticed how much stronger my legs are and how much better my balance is when I went skiing and was able to stand on one leg to take my snow pants off.
- I haven't needed my mid-afternoon energy drink because I've had plenty of energy!
- I went out for drinks with friends and had no problem sticking to the 2-drink limit I'd set for myself.
- I asked for weights for my birthday, which is something I never would have done before!
- I increased the weights for my chest press to 25 lb and could still do 10 reps.

Once you've decided on the metrics you want to use for your progress updates, decide on the frequency with which you'll collect that data. For photos and measurements, I recommend weekly or twice-a-month updates. Your measurements and photos won't change drastically from one week to the next but getting practice at collecting the data will ensure that you're measuring the same sites or taking photos with the same lighting and angles so that your data is accurate and useful for comparison purposes. It makes sense to pair your weekly progress updates with your weekly life admin so that you can use the data you're collecting to help you reflect on the previous week and to set goals for the upcoming one.

Metrics like health markers your doctor will run labs to test may only be done every three to six months, while others like mood and performance are easy to track weekly. I recommend keeping a running Non-Scale Victory list in your phone so you can update it anytime you notice a win.

Determining Your Progress Metrics

Which metrics will you track?

How frequently will you track them?

Where will you record this data? (Digitally, paper calendar, etc.)

Why are these important to you?

WEEKLY LIFE ADMIN

Getting in the habit of doing weekly "life admin" made Lou's life exponentially better, as it will yours.

She was usually so burned out from the work week that she wanted weekends to be an opportunity to shut her brain off, think as little as possible, and just chill. Except that they were generally packed with birthday parties, sports games, visits with her parents, chores, and a million other things that seem to monopolize every waking second. Before she knew it, her alarm was going off way too early on Monday morning, and she was off to the races for yet another chaotic week.

Although she was in the habit of planning dinners and grocery shopping (she wouldn't survive the week without it), she was struggling to stay on top of which kid needed to be where and on what day and time, which days were the longest or busiest, her own meeting schedule, and any appointments or obligation outside the normal blur of the week.

When I suggested weekly "life admin" to her, she was resistant; she genuinely felt like she didn't have time for one more thing.

I explained that just a few minutes once a week would be plenty for her to go into the week with a realistic plan she was confident she could execute in the midst of the chaos. She knew that the current cycle wasn't going to break itself and that she needed to do things differently if she wanted to get the weight off and her life back.

Once she started, she realized that even that small time investment made her work week so much smoother and more productive, and she wasn't feeling so exhausted and frazzled by the time the weekend rolled around. Since she was getting more done during the week, things weren't getting pushed to the weekend, which gave her more time to relax and enjoy her life. Being better rested put her in a better headspace about tackling the week ahead, and her successes grew from there.

Here's how you can build the habit of "life admin" into your own life:

Add a 30-minute recurring weekly event to your calendar for every Sunday morning (or whatever day and time makes the most sense for your life). Once you're in the habit, you may only need 15 minutes or less, but give yourself time to be a beginner.

Ideally, create a quiet and uninterrupted environment for yourself so you can concentrate, but if you find yourself doing "life admin" while sitting in the bleachers at a baseball game, so be it. Done is better than perfect.

I encourage you to make copies of the worksheets in your book portal (www.estheravant.com/book-portal-signup) or designate a notebook for your weekly self-check-ins.

Not only will it be super helpful during your monthly and quarterly check-ins, but you will love to be able to look back on the early days of your journey once you get further along. There's no better way to see how far you've come than to read, in your own words, what you were proud of, and what tripped you up when you first started.

First, you'll reflect on the week that has just ended:

Weekly Recap

Using the data you're collecting, including less-tangible data such as your energy levels or mood, allows you the opportunity to develop awareness, get curious, make connections and discover patterns, and experiment with strategies that will help you lose weight and keep it off. For example, looking back at your food log to see which specific foods or combinations helped you feel your best and have the most energy can help you tweak your diet to have more days like that.

Developing the skill of reflecting can help if you find yourself falling short of your weekly behavior goals. Rather than thinking you're just lacking discipline or willpower, you'll likely realize that but there are minor obstacles with easy solutions. When my client Monica realized that not wanting to put on workout clothes was the actual reason she was skipping her workouts, she started exercising in her pajamas and she rarely misses one now!

Reflecting on your previous week's efforts better allows you to take compassionate ownership of your results. If you're finding yourself feeling discouraged by lack of progress one month, but you look back and realize that you rated your efforts between a five and a seven on a scale of one to ten each week, you know right away that you just need to turn your effort dials up, rather than going into a tailspin thinking something is wrong with you.

The more detail you include in your check-ins, the more useful this meeting with yourself will be. This information is also invaluable for looking at trends over longer periods of time during your monthly and quarterly meetings. (For example, there's no reason to be alarmed if your sleep and energy were low one week, especially if you're noticing it corresponded with your period, but if you look back at the end of the month and realize sleep and energy were low *most* of the month or quarter, that's something to explore.)

Below you'll find a short version of a weekly check-in you can use to give yourself a big picture view of your week and help you set goals. In your book portal (http://www.estheravant.com/book-portal-signup), you'll find worksheets with the exact questions I ask my clients during their weekly check-ins, which goes more in depth in all the same areas. Either version works great and will help you get a comprehensive look at all of the components of your lifestyle that can impact your weight loss. The important thing is that you just start grooving the habit of doing your weekly life admin,. so choose whichever format you prefer.

You might be a little overwhelmed at the idea of starting—that's okay! The first couple times you do anything new can feel a bit clunky, but after a few sessions, you'll find your groove and your life admin probably won't take more than a handful of minutes.

Progress Update

Record any metrics you tracked this week to help you gauge your progress (scale weight, measurements, photos, etc.)

Weekly Reflection Overview

Write down your Wins this week (this can be scale victories, measurements, Non-Scale Victories (NSVs), compliments, Personal Records (PRs), following through on commitments to yourself, ANYTHING you're proud of).

What didn't go well this week and what can you learn from those challenges? (The more thoughtfully you can answer, the better. For example, "Have a go-to backup plan of what to order at the restaurant near work" is a more useful takeaway than "Don't forget my lunch next time.")

Exercise "Big Rocks"

Make some notes on your daily steps, strength workouts, rest days, and any additional exercise you did this week. How do these compare to the goals you set for this week? If you fell short of your goals, reflect on why.

On a scale of 1-10, how happy are you with your exercise EFFORTS this week? Why did you choose that number?

Nutrition "Big Rocks"

Make some notes on your nutrition this week to include your calories, protein, and fiber (if you're tracking your food), as well as any additional nutrition habits you're working on. How do these compare to the goals you set for this week? If you fell short of your goals, reflect on why.

On a scale of 1-10, how happy are you with your nutrition EFFORTS this week? Why did you choose that number?

Lifestyle Factors

If you have a period, where are you in your cycle? What sort of impact do you think that may have had on your mood, energy, appetite, results, etc., this week?

How many hours of sleep did you average per night this week?

On a scale of 1-10, how would you rate your energy levels this week?

On a scale of 1-10, how would you rate your stress levels this week? (If applicable) What strategies did you use to reduce it or cope with it?

How supported did you feel by your support system this week? Is there anyone you can reach out to next week for more support (if needed)?

Upcoming Week

It's important to adjust your weekly behavior goals based on both the data you have from the previous week *and* what's going on in your life the upcoming week. Without being intentional and planning ahead, you run the risk of blindly setting goals that look good on paper, but then falling short and damaging your self-trust with each passing week. Prioritizing weekly goal-setting sessions gives you the opportunity to set realistic goals you're confident you can accomplish, collect wins, and build momentum to keep going.

For Lou, this meant knowing that when she had back-to-back meetings that led straight into her daughter's softball games, she wouldn't be able to work out in the afternoon or evening like she preferred, so she would instead work out in the morning. It wasn't her preference (in fact, she *hated* it and couldn't fathom how anyone could be a morning person and do it regularly), but she did it because she saw the value of being consistent with her workouts, so having to do it early was better than not doing it at all. She knew that it was the small, daily decisions like these that would help her reach her weight-loss goals.

In the beginning, it will benefit you to be as specific as possible with your goals, which might mean putting workouts, grocery shopping, meal planning, meal prep, bedtime, and social media-free time all in your calendar. As you develop routines that support your weight loss and you're in the habit of doing the "Big Rocks" consistently, you may not need the same level of detail in order to ensure you follow through.

When setting weekly goals, it's important to remember that curveballs are a part of life and sometimes you'll make a great plan that ends up going sideways in ways you couldn't have anticipated. When this happens, it's equally important to practice the skills of being flexible and unattached to *exactly* when or how things get done but committed to *getting* them done most of the time, because it's the small, day-to-day choices that create the lasting weight loss you're after.

Compassionate ownership will help you in the event you don't reach your goals:

If you fall short of your goals on occasion for reasons out of your control, lean on your self-compassion, look for the lesson, and move on.

If you're *consistently* falling short of your workout, nutrition, or lifestyle goals more than two weeks in a row, take ownership of figuring out why and how to adjust accordingly.

Weekly Goal Setting

Exercise "Big Rocks" (Steps, Strength, Rest)

Do you have a daily step goal this week? If so, what?

Will you strength train this week? If so, how many times, which days/times, and what will you do?

When will you take rest/active recovery days? What will you do during them?

What, if any, exercise goals do you have outside of the "Big Rocks"?

Nutrition "Big Rocks" (Calories, Protein, Fiber)

Are you tracking your food this week? If so, are you focusing on all the "Big Rocks" or just one to two of them? If not, what are your nutrition goals this week?

What, if any, nutrition goals do you have outside of the "Big Rocks"?

Lifestyle Goals

Do you have goals related to sleep or stress management this week? If so, what? (how many hours of sleep, what time you'll go to bed or wake up, what stress management strategies you'll implement and when, etc.,)

What other, if any, lifestyle-related goals do you have this week?

Support & Accountability

Weekly "life admin" is a good opportunity to think about what kind of support or help you need for the upcoming week, especially because *making* a plan doesn't necessarily mean you will want to do the things at their scheduled times. How will *you* prepare for when your short-term desires and long-term goals are at odds and remind yourself that you want the outcome of following your plan and doing the "Big Rocks" consistently? Who can you enlist to help you follow through on your goals?

Whether or not you're working with a professional, it's still important to have an outlet for support, guidance, and accountability questions and to communicate what you need from your advisory board of support people. As we talked about in Chapter 9, your spouse, kids, coworkers, friends, and even people you don't know in real life can all help support you. Although they can't read your mind, if you clearly ask for what you need, they'll likely be happy to provide it.

For Lou, this meant giving her husband a very specific grocery list to pick up on the way home from work, having her kids each pick out a dinner recipe, and asking a coworker to ping her to make sure she was eating her lunch.

If you have exercise- or nutrition-related questions, writing them out can help you get clear on exactly what information you're looking for and where to find it. Without being specific about the challenge and what you need to overcome it, it's easy for small obstacles like, "Squats hurt my knees" to turn into, "I guess I can't work out." Once you have clarity on what you need to know ("How can I modify squats so that my knees don't hurt?"), you'll be better able to find answers. They may be a quick Google search away (be careful with sources), or they may help you realize that you would benefit from the guidance of a professional and having specific examples of what you would like help with will help guide you in what kind support and accountability you need.

Questions

What workout- or nutrition-related questions or concerns do you have right now?

Where will you get answers to those questions?

In addition to getting answers to any questions that you have, it's also important to anticipate obstacles that may come up throughout the week and have a plan for overcoming them so that you can be consistent with the "Big Rocks." Here are some ways you can practice doing that:

Anticipating Challenges & Finding Solutions

Visualize getting a calendar alert and really not wanting to do the workout of whatever you have scheduled at that time. What will you do?

How will you remind yourself that this seemingly inconsequential task is important enough for reaching your goals that you'll do it even if you don't feel like it? What conversation will you have with yourself to help you follow through?

What excuses is your brain likely to come up with and how will you overcome those?

What solutions or contingency plans do you need to have handy for the inevitable obstacles that pop up and prevent things from going according to plan A? (There are always more solutions than there are excuses, but you have to train yourself to find them).

Whose help do you need to enlist this week? Who will help support you and hold you accountable? How?

Daily Adjustments

Setting aside a few minutes each evening to reflect on the previous day and review the plan for the upcoming day will help you make the small adjustments that can help the week go more smoothly. With time, you'll likely be able to do this in your head, but in the beginning, it can be helpful to have a little bit of designated time to sit down and do it.

If you're tracking your food, this is a great opportunity to track in advance based on your meal plan for the day and cut down on how much time you spend doing it in the moment.

Just taking a minute to think, "How did this morning's early wakeup go? What could I do to make that smoother? Do I want to tweak anything about tomorrow?" can help you find your groove faster than if you were only checking in with yourself once a week.

Figuring out what "life admin" looks like for *you* will be an ever-evolving process. Maybe your exercise "Big Rocks" need to be planned very specifically and include back-up plans, but you realize you only need a loose meal plan because you like giving yourself options to choose between based on how you're feeling that day. Maybe you've been consistent enough with workouts to know you'll find a way to get those in, but the nutrition "Big Rocks" necessitate a more specific plan.

Daily Reflection & Plan Tweaks

How did today go? What went well? What challenged you? How will you avoid or overcome those challenges in the future?

Is the plan you created for the exercise and nutrition "Big Rocks" for tomorrow still feasible or do you need to tweak anything?

MONTHLY

Every month I host a reflection and goal-setting call in our client community as an opportunity for our ladies to pause and publicly celebrate their wins that might otherwise go unnoticed. They also have the opportunity to share challenges and get the support of other women who can relate.

The skill of anticipating obstacles will help you be prepared for predictable occurrences that you previously hadn't had the awareness to notice, and brainstorming solutions will help you think in a more solutions-oriented way.

For example, June could mark the first month of travel soccer season, which means long weekend days spent out of the house in the car or sitting in the hot sun on the sidelines. Instead of being caught off guard and running through the drive-thru every weekend (sometimes more than once!), you know you'll be better off if you set aside some time to batch prep some basic ingredients to bring some meals with you.

Monthly "life admin" helps you anticipate how your needs are going to change in the coming weeks so you can make a plan that will help you stay consistent despite those changes.

Consider inviting your spouse, kids, or friends to participate so you can celebrate one another and help each other troubleshoot obstacles.

Here are the questions my clients consider each month:

Monthly Reflection

What were your behavior goals this month? (Like number of workouts, days tracked, etc.)

What were your outcomes/results and what did you do to get those results? (Example: lost 5 lb and 7 inches. Completed 95% of workouts, tracked 100% of the time, etc.)

What wins did you have besides the scale or measurements?

What have you done to celebrate your accomplishments?

What did you learn this month? How have you grown or shifted?

What were your most common thoughts & feelings this month?

What went well this month that you want to continue doing next month?

What didn't go well this month that you want to stop doing next month?

Monthly Goal Setting

What goals are you setting for next month?

What actions will you take to reach those goals?

What changes do you anticipate this month that could potentially prevent you from reaching those goals? For each obstacle, list at least one solution.

What will you do to celebrate your successes throughout and at the end of this month?

QUARTERLY

Your quarterly check-ins are a great opportunity to revisit your yearly goals since the annual planning you outlined in the previous chapter can be hard to do when you aren't sure what is in store for you months down the road. As time passes, new events and obligations will pop up. Add them to your calendar during your quarterly "life admin" meetings so you can map out your surge and cruise opportunities for the next three to six months and adjust your plans accordingly.

Quarterly meetings are an opportunity to celebrate your wins and accomplishments of the past few months. It's likely you're spending most of your time thinking about how far you still have to go and are overlooking the wins along the way that make the journey feel more enjoyable. Taking time to reflect and appreciate yourself for everything you've done so far helps you build the confidence to keep going.

Lastly, quarterly "life admin" is a chance to reflect on opportunities you have to learn and grow.

Some questions to ask yourself:

Quarterly Reflection

Are there any outcome goals you've already accomplished?

Are your remaining outcome goals still important to you? Are there any you've decided are no longer a priority?

Has your "why" changed at all, or are you still just as committed as before? (If you're not feeling committed, spend some time going through the 5 Whys exercise to get clear on why it's important *now* for you to keep going.)

How consistently have you been doing the "Big Rocks"? (Tracking a variety of metrics as we'll discuss in the Weekly "Life Admin" section will make it very easy to look back at a quarter's worth of data to help you notice trends and patterns).

How much progress have you made since your previous quarterly meeting?

What skills or tools have you developed over the last quarter?

How does your progress compare to what you were expecting?

How confident are you feeling about your strategy to continue making progress?

What challenges did you encounter?

What skills or tools do you want to develop to overcome them?

Like all the skills and tools we've discussed so far and the lifestyle- and mindset-focused ones (like overcoming self-sabotage and time management that we'll cover in the next chapter), if you're consistent and committed to the practice of doing "life admin," you'll have plenty of opportunities to experiment and make it work for you.

CHAPTER 13

FILLING YOUR TOOLBOX

My dad is a carpenter and woodworker who built our house with his own two calloused, banged up hands. One of my favorite childhood photos is of me around age four, smiling into the camera with long, tangled hair, a big apron, and holding a small hammer I'd just pulled out of the wooden toolbox he'd made just for me.

He loved scouring the classified section of the weekly paper for any ads that had tools listed in the five-line description and perusing garage sales for just the tool he was looking for.

His tools overflowed the giant Stihl toolbox on wheels he had in the garage, and it didn't matter the job, he'd be able to find the right tool for it (sometimes more easily than others). He was already skilled with most of them, and he was also confident that he could learn how to use a new one or find a new use for a familiar one.

As you know from Chapter 10, tools aren't just for carpentry: they're devices or implements that carry out particular functions. Just like my dad, your job is to develop a robust set of tools so that no matter what the job (obstacle), you have a tool for it or are confident you can find and learn how to use one.

This chapter is all about starting to fill up your personal Obstacle Toolbox.

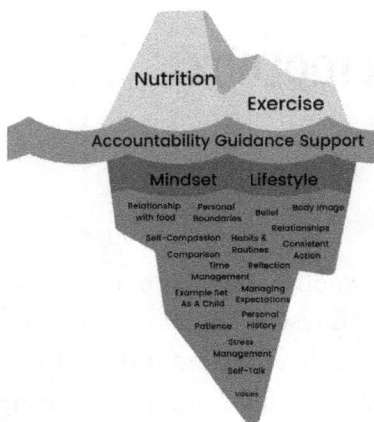

Nutrition

Exercise

Accountability Guidance Support

Mindset   Lifestyle

Relationship with food   Personal Boundaries   Belief   Body image
Relationships
Self-Compassion   Habits & Routines   Consistent Action
Comparison
Time Management   Reflection
Example Set As A Child   Managing Expectations
Personal History
Patience
Stress Management
Self-Talk
Values

By now, hopefully you understand why just being told what to do and following the rules never leads to the lasting weight loss you're after. Your life and body are far too dynamic for there to be a one-size-fits-all "solution."

Taking compassionate ownership (Chapter 10) helps you recognize the skills and tools that *you* need to develop and have the willingness to be a beginner and actually put in the work to master them. This is "the work" that most women don't do.

There **will** be challenges along the way, whether you are just beginning your weight-loss journey, transitioning to maintenance, or somewhere in between. That's fine. Your self-awareness and growth mindset allow you to identify and overcome new obstacles anytime they arise.

While there's no standard set of skills and tools for you to collect like Pokémon cards and then be done, there's also nothing you can't learn, do, or figure out, and each challenge you face is just an opportunity to practice developing a new skill or tool—and with it, confidence—that will serve you then and in the future. Be curious and willing to go where the journey takes you, even if it's an unexpected direction.

As you practice learning and mastering the exercise and nutrition "Big Rocks," you'll see that it's much less about the specific exercises or meals full of "superfoods," and more about discovering the broader lifestyle obstacles that are preventing you from showing up for yourself consistently. The skills and tools we're talking about in this chapter are the ones that address the beneath-the-surface obstacles affecting your mindset and lifestyle that can have a big indirect impact on your ability to lose weight and keep it off.

Remember that all skills and tools take time and practice to master. Just like when I first started using that little hammer to "help" my dad and mostly whacked my thumb over and over until I finally figured it out, you can't expect yourself to master anything new without continued practice. Allow yourself to be a beginner, an imperfect human, and work on honing your skills over time.

The rest of this chapter is devoted to some of the common lifestyle and mindset challenges I see most women facing. It is not a comprehensive list but provides a broad overview of areas to consider for yourself. Working with a professional such as a therapist, life coach, or a program like mine can help you deep-dive into the issues that will benefit you the most. This chapter includes some preliminary tips for how to start developing the skills and tools that will help you address lifestyle- and mindset-related obstacles that are making your weight loss harder to maintain or achieve in the first place. These are especially important to look to help you uncover underlying reasons why you're having a hard time being consistent with the "Big Rocks."

LIFESTYLE
Shaping Your Environment

Most of us don't realize just how much our environment impacts the choices we make. You mindlessly grab a handful of trail mix from the pantry because it's right there when you open it to get out the pasta for dinner. You go out for lunch when you're at the office because there's a restaurant in the same building that everyone else goes to. You toss candy into your cart at the store because it's right there at the checkout.

Changing your environment can eliminate willpower battles.

As mentioned, not bringing "trigger foods" into the house or storing them in out-of-the-way places can make a huge difference in mindless or emotional eating. Taking a different route to or from work can break the habit of getting a high-calorie coffee and muffin before work or swinging through the drive-thru on the way home. Bringing your dumbbells or yoga mat into the living room or changing before you get home from work can make it that much easier to actually get your workout in.

If this feels relevant to you, consider keeping a journal throughout the next week of ways that your environment is or isn't supporting your goals and start making small changes to have fewer obstacles in your path.

Setting Boundaries

Boundaries define what behaviors, interactions, or experiences are acceptable for you. Losing weight will likely require setting boundaries with other people—and yourself.

Interpersonal boundaries might include asking loved ones not to comment on your body, engage in diet talk around you, or critique your food choices.

According to Melissa Urban, author of *The Book of Boundaries*, there are three steps to setting boundaries:

1. Identify the need for one. (This requires noticing how other people's behavior impacts you).

2. Set it using clear, direct, and kind language. When you're done talking, the person should know exactly where your limit is and how to avoid crossing it. Don't go into it assuming the worst; odds are, most people with whom you're setting boundaries will respect them.

3. If a boundary is being crossed, you owe it to yourself to follow through on upholding the consequence.

When it comes to setting self-boundaries, make sure you're framing them in a way that upholding them feels like an act of self-care rather than a punishment. For example, if you're setting a boundary around your morning phone use, in the moment it can feel like there is no consequence if you don't uphold it; after all, you're the only person who will know or be impacted. But there *are* consequences, and you're *not* necessarily the only person affected.

Starting your morning off with doom scrolling means squandering your opportunity to have a productive or relaxed morning and instead being rushed and irritable when you finally get out of bed and generally feeling like you're starting the day off on the wrong foot.

Focusing on the freedom the boundary affords you will help you uphold it when you're tempted not to. That freedom could look like a leisurely start to the day during which you can work out, eat breakfast, or even just enjoy a cup of coffee before the kids wake up. Upholding that phone boundary makes the difference between starting the day being proactive rather than reactive.

When it comes to setting boundaries with yourself, give yourself grace and keep trying, even when it feels hard and know that you CAN trust yourself and you ARE worth keeping promises to.

Improving Time Management

Time is the only asset you can't get back. When you don't have a plan for where to spend it, it gets spent for you on things you may not want or care about.

Work and family may naturally dictate a lot of your schedule, leaving you with nothing left over for yourself. Being intentional about how you spend your time (specifically carving out time for YOU) will help you lose weight and create a lifestyle that allows you to keep it off. Put appointments in your calendar for the things that are important to reach your goals, like your workouts, grocery shopping, meal planning, bedtime, and therapy. Prioritizing yourself *isn't* selfish and, in fact, ripples out and benefits everyone around you.

If you're not sure where your time is going, do a time audit where you document exactly what you're doing in 15 to 30-minute increments to better understand where your time is being allocated. You can tell a lot about a person based on where they spend their time, so if the audit reveals that your current breakdown isn't in alignment with your values and goals, you can start making changes from there.

Overcoming Emotional & Mindless Eating

Practically, there are a few things you can do about foods you have a hard time moderating:

- Stop bringing them into your home or work environments. If they're not there, you can't eat them.

- If you HAVE to have those foods around because of other people, buy single-serving packages or portion them out as soon as you bring them home.

- Store temptations out of sight and hard to reach. The more obstacles between, the better. This won't stop you 100% of the time (I've climbed on the counter to get the peanut butter from the top of the fridge), but it builds in a series of opportunities to pause, notice what you're doing, and decide if you want to continue.

- Make the foods you *want* to be eating as easy to access as possible, such as washing and chopping produce and storing them on the counter or front and center in the fridge.

These tools will help you break the patterns of automatic behavior, but it's also important to address the root issue that's causing you to eat emotionally or mindlessly (if there is one).

Journaling or keeping a behavior awareness journal can help you connect the behavior to its trigger. With that awareness, you will be able to anticipate and avoid the cycle with healthier coping mechanisms like exercise, journaling, yoga, meditation, posting in a FB group, calling someone, working on a project, reading, doing a puzzle, or whatever makes sense for you.

Learning to Not Be Peer Pressured

As I mentioned in Chapter 2, modern society makes it hard to maintain a healthy weight. Behaviors that are "normal" for most people are largely incompatible with reaching and staying at a healthy weight. Are you willing to live a lifestyle that other people might think is weird or might make you stand out, for the satisfaction, health, confidence, and happiness of achieving what few people do?

You can learn to rise above peer pressure (overt or perceived) and feel comfortable communicating your needs, upholding your boundaries, and not caring if other people don't understand or support your choices. Your wants and needs are allowed to trump other people's preferences and opinions a lot of the time. For example, it's okay to decline another glass of wine after reaching the limit you've set for yourself, no matter how much your best friend pouts and begs you to have one more. It might feel easier to give in, but what *she* wants isn't more important than what you want, and other people's reactions say more about them than they do about you. Practice letting them roll off your back as you remain committed to reaching your weight-loss goals and becoming the person you want to be.

Creating Routine Where It's Lacking (weekends, travel)

Most of us find it easier to be consistent with the "Big Rocks" during the work week when we have built-in structure that helps shape our days. Disruptions to routine—even recurring ones like weekends—are generally the times we start to waver. In order to achieve weight loss that lasts, it's important to figure out how to stay consistent and committed regardless of location or day of the week.

"Life admin" as covered in Chapter 12 can help you anticipate and plan for disruptions to your routines. For example, knowing that you'll have long days out of the house this weekend will help you be better prepared with a plan for food to bring with you and when you'll get in your steps or workouts.

One way to help yourself stay consistent is to look at the "anchors" (small, foundational habits) that help you stay committed to your weight-loss goals during the week and figure out how to replicate them in some way during the less structured times. This can be something like doing some form of movement in the mornings, even on weekends or away from home or eating your normal breakfast even on vacation.

Most people can see that they're more successful with some structure but are reluctant to create it for fear of being boxed in. The key is to be committed to the goal but flexible in your approach. Habits, routines, and structure are simply ways to give yourself parameters that help you be consistent with the "Big Rocks." With time and experimentation, you'll find your personal sweet spot where you're getting the best of both worlds.

When it comes to traveling, remember that your effort dials can always be adjusted to account for the other demands on your time and energy. Coming up with what I like to call travel "Bare-Ass Minimums" (BAMs) can help you turn your dials down to something reasonable given your circumstances, while still showing up for yourself and your goals. This could look like committing to a few ten-minute body weight workouts in your hotel room on the same mornings you normally workout at home, adjusting your step goal to account for sitting in work meetings all day, or capping the number of alcoholic drinks you'll have on the trip. Continuing to groove the "Big Rock" habits in small ways will benefit you and help make for a smoother transition back into your routines when you return home.

MINDSET

The importance of your mindset and mental state really can't be overstated, in general or as they relate to your ability to lose weight and keep it off. How and what you think impacts *everything* and would be impossible for me to cover fully in this book.

The following section is intended to help you understand and begin to address common mindset-related challenges that many women face during their weight-loss journeys. It does not, and should not, replace working with a mental health professional such as a therapist to help you unpack and work through any psychological issues that are holding you back from living your healthiest, happiest, and most confident life.

Improving Your Relationship With The Scale

The scale is only one small piece of the picture when it comes to weight loss, health, and happiness. It will never tell you the full story and should always be used in conjunction with other indicators of progress so you don't overlook the (more meaningful) progress that's happening elsewhere.

Can a scale be useful? Sure. But using it is optional. If it makes you feel like a failure or is the catalyst for self-sabotage when you're not seeing progress as quickly as you'd like, consider taking a break from it. When I was pregnant with my son, I knew it would be mentally tough for me to see the number increase week after week for the better part of a year, so I chose to stop using the scale. More than five years later, I still don't know what I weigh, and I've never been healthier, happier, or more confident in my body.

I have clients who have been successful with using it daily, every few days, once a week, or not at all. Give yourself the opportunity to experiment with different frequencies to see how they feel. The most value it provides is to look at trends over time, so the sweet spot for many of my clients has been three times per week and using an app like HappyScale that shows you the trend of your progress.

Make sure you're also tracking other metrics that are important to you, like measurements, photos, how your clothes are fitting, and an ongoing list of non-scale victories to help remind you that the true meaningful progress you're after has little to do with numbers.

Processing Body Image/Weight-Related Issues From Childhood

Many of my clients have realized that their body image and self-worth issues stem all the way back to childhood. They grew up watching their mothers do diet after diet, pick themselves apart in the mirror, were dragged along to WW meetings from age ten, and heard loud and clear that thin = good and fat = bad. Those beliefs are still inside many of us, and of *course* they're having an impact on our present and future.

As the squeeze generation (both raising kids and taking care of aging parents), a lot of women feel caught in the middle: resentful of their mothers (who may still be struggling with their weight/body image issues), unhappy and uncomfortable in their own bodies, and concerned about what their own kids are picking up on. You are probably doing everything in your power to avoid passing that trauma on to your own children, which can make losing weight even more difficult.

Professional help in the form of therapy or life coaching can help you work through these experiences and emotions, see your value and worth independent of your size, and help you repair, or at least move forward from, the childhood relationship with your mother.

Rebuilding Your Reputation With Yourself

If you're in the position of having spent years setting and falling short of your goals, you've trained yourself to believe that what you say doesn't matter because you're not going to follow through, anyway. It's not too late to prove to yourself that you *are* trustworthy and reliable.

You come through when someone else needs you, whether that's a last-minute project, costume, baked goods for your kids, a ride to the airport for a friend, or taking on more responsibility at work.

It's likely that the only time you don't do what you say you'll do is when you think *you're* the only person impacted. But are you really the only one? No! When you're in the habit of following through on your commitments to yourself, everyone in your life gets a better version of you, as well.

The steps for earning back your self-trust are:

- Forgive yourself for the past and wipe the slate clean.
- Set small daily goals that you're confident you can accomplish.
- Follow through on those goals at least 85% of the time (enlist your support system to help with accountability).

- ive yourself time to heal and start seeing yourself as someone who's reliable, whether someone else is looking or not.

Overcoming Self-Sabotage

The difference between occasional indulging and self-sabotage is that self-sabotaging behavior creates problems in your daily life and interferes with your long-term goals.

Occasionally overeating like you might find yourself doing on vacation may not actually be a problem or hinder your results, so that would be an example of just living in the "messy middle" rather than self-sabotage. If you frequently eat your feelings when you're frustrated with the scale or use food to reward yourself when it's cooperating, that could be self-sabotage. Anything that impacts your results (or lack thereof) or causes mental turmoil would fit into this category.

The frequency and severity with which you engage in— and the outcome of—the behavior is what determines whether or not it's self-sabotage.

Self-sabotaging actions are driven by feelings that are caused by thoughts, though you may not yet be aware of those thoughts or feelings.

If you're engaging in a behavior you're not happy with but don't know the root cause of it, keeping a behavior awareness journal can help you make the connections between your environment, company, thoughts, and actions. Start to question whether these surroundings, people, thoughts, feelings, and behaviors are serving you or if you'd like to change them (you can!). From there, it'll be easier for you to see patterns or triggers that you can work on addressing so the current cycle of self-sabotage doesn't continue.

Keep in mind that self-sabotage is just a learned behavior that you've chosen repeatedly, so breaking the habit is just a matter of intentionally and repeatedly choosing different thoughts that inspire different actions.

Once you're aware of the circumstances that typically precede an instance of self-sabotage an "if/then statement" can help you pre-commit to the new behavior you want to take in the future. For example, "if I have a stressful day at work and really want a glass of wine to unwind, I'll remind myself that alcohol actually ends up making me feel worse and I'll have a mocktail and call a friend to vent, instead."

Behavior Awareness Prompts

Think about where you were, with whom, doing what, and how you were feeling in the hours and minutes leading up to a self-sabotage episode to help you identify the root cause so you can work on breaking the cycle:

What were you doing before?

Where were you?

Who were you with?

How were you feeling?

What were you thinking?

Where are the opportunities to avoid this in the future?

What new thoughts could help you break the current cycle of self-sabotage?

If those were your new thoughts, how would your actions change?

What "if/then statements" would help you pre-commit to the actions you want to take?

Improving Self-Talk & The Stories We Tell Ourselves

Imagine waking up every morning for years and writing nasty messages to your daughter or friend on the bathroom mirror about what a "fat, unlovable, worthless person" she is. You would never do that!

But you may have looked at yourself in the mirror every morning for years and said similar things about yourself, and you've come to believe that they're true.

The stories we tell ourselves about ourselves, other people, and the world shape how we think and feel about ourselves, what we think we can do, who we think we are, and what we deserve of. We show up as the person we think we are.

Things you believe to be true (everything from "I'm just not a morning person" to "No one will ever love me") are not irrefutable *facts*, just thoughts you've had so many times that you *believe them to be true*.

Here are three questions to help you retire the old "soundtracks" (beliefs that are really just repetitive thoughts), from the book *Soundtracks: The Surprising Solution to Overthinking* by Jon Acuff:

- Is it true? Look for evidence to help you dispute it.

- Is it kind? Does this belief make you feel good or bad?

- Is it helpful? When you think this thought, does it help you move forward toward your goals or is it keeping you stuck, perpetuating you getting the same outcome that you always have?

Physical changes won't change how you feel about yourself; smaller doesn't equal happier. Making lasting changes to how you *look* means also addressing how you *feel* about yourself. Believing that you are worthy and valuable *as you are* is the only way to make changes that stick.

To take the power away from your inner critic:

- Give her a name (like Bitter Betty or Mean Martha)

- Speak in the third person, as though you're a TV narrator ("Esther is eating peanut butter because she's lonely.") This distance between your thoughts and reactions allows you to question whether your thoughts are *really* true. What are the facts? What evidence do you have? What evidence do you have that the opposite might be true?

- Use the "loved one" litmus test where you ask yourself what you would say to your daughter or best friend and how you would respond to negative comments she was making about herself. This can help you relearn how to speak to yourself like someone you love.

The following journaling prompts will help you understand your current thoughts and beliefs as well as develop some new, more positive ones to try on going forward. If you're having a hard time coming up with new positive beliefs that feel true, work on just removing the negativity from your current beliefs and making them more neutral first. For example, instead of referring to your "flabby" arms, just say arms.

You may also want to refer back to the Breakup Letter and Postcard From Your Future Self exercises from Chapter 6.

Journaling Prompts

What things do you say to yourself?

What beliefs/stories do you have about yourself based on the things you tell yourself?

How have those beliefs/stories served you in the past?

How would you *like* to see yourself?

What new beliefs/stories about yourself will you try on? (Repeating these mantras to yourself in the mirror every day can be incredibly powerful!)

CONCLUSION

Now you know the formula to lose weight, keep it off, and live a healthier, happier, and more confident life than you've imagined. Here is where you get to practice making it work for YOU. That's how I want you to think about the work that starts now: practice. You're applying. You're experimenting. You're learning. You're iterating. And it's all a part of the process.

You can't mess this up. When you feel like you have, that's just a sign to practice treating yourself with compassion, get curious, take ownership, and lean on your support system.

While I don't believe that we ever really "arrive" or have it all figured out (when it comes to weight loss, health, or *anything* really), there will be undeniable signs that you're not where you used to be and when you notice them, it'll feel amazing.

I had one such realization the other day.

Instead of waking up at the crack of dawn to drive to a local gym and do at least an hour of cardio before anyone else in my family woke up, I started my morning after sunrise with a short dumbbell strength workout on the deck overlooking the river at my dad's. These days, it's not a priority for me to spend a lot of time inside a gym when I know I can get in an effective workout with minimal equipment and time. Then I did a ten-minute yoga class, something my son likes doing with me (as long as I let him pick the class). I drank the 24 ounces of water I like to have to front-load my day and ate my "go to" breakfast of eggs, veggies, potatoes, and avocado that I look forward to every day and know gives me an appropriate number of calories, protein, and fiber to fuel me for hours. I didn't stress about the unknowns in store later in the day or try to "save" all my calories just in case. All of this came easily and without relying on motivation or discipline. I didn't need to think about these things, because they're just part of who I am now.

Knowing it would be a warm, sunny day, the local blueberry festival seemed like the perfect place to spend the afternoon. My son and I could be outside, walking around, both having fun.

It didn't even cross my mind to do extra cardio to make up for "overindulging" on fair food. It didn't even cross my mind to be anxious about not being able to control myself around all the many temptations.

When we were offered free blueberry pie with ice cream, I decided, "Yes, making this memory feels like a worthy indulgence to me." And also, "Splitting a piece of pie with my son doesn't mean I've ruined anything. I don't need to throw in the towel for the rest of the day. I don't need to use this as an excuse to eat everything else that I come across. I don't need to make up for it by skipping dinner later or working out extra hard tomorrow. I can savor it, take in my surroundings, and appreciate this moment."

The way we talk to ourselves matters. Being mindful and aware of what we're doing and thinking matters. These allowed me to notice when I felt satisfied and stop then, rather than

ACKNOWLEDGEMENTS

Thank you to all of my former and current coaching clients. To the OGs who saw my potential before I felt like I knew what I was doing and entrusted me to help guide you while I was figuring out this whole Business Owner thing. To the long-term clients who've seen the ongoing evolution of EA Coaching. To the clients who continue to check in and give me life updates, even years after graduating from coaching. You've allowed me to have the best job in the world and if not for your influence, I wouldn't have had a book to write. Thank you for letting me be a part of your lives.

To my team at EA Coaching: Amber, Emilia, Jenny, Lauren, Lindsay, Rachel. Thank you for being a part of my vision. I know each and every one of you cares about our clients and mission just as much as I do.

To Meg: From that first, "I don't know what I'm doing but can you help?" conversation, you've been my rock. It's a pleasure learning, growing, and evolving with you, and I'm so, so proud of who we've both become and what we've created and will continue to create together.

To everyone who has helped me go from "Maybe I'd like to write a book one day" to a real book: Lou for being the first "real" author I knew and for being supportive and encouraging when I mentioned writing a book.

My first coach, Jessica: The AUTHORity Blueprint is exactly what I needed to go from a jumbled mess in my brain to a rough draft.

My second coach, Sara: Thought Leader Academy helped me realize that the only difference between me and "real" authors is that they've written a book and I hadn't . . . yet.

My editor, Hannah: The improvements in this book from our first session to our last are incredible. Without you, this book just wouldn't be nearly as good.

To all the friends, peers, even strangers to whom I mentioned I was writing a book and didn't laugh me out of town (so, all of you, that never happened). Thank you. I was never once made to feel like I had no business writing a book, and I can't say how much that boosted my confidence in actually making it happen.

To my beta readers, Beth, Jaime, Jennifer, Joanne, Nicky: You guys were AMAZING! I couldn't have asked for more thorough and thoughtful feedback. I hope you can see the ways this book is better because of your influence.

To Dad: You've always been my #1 supporter, from being the only person reading my early blogs to sharing every Facebook post I've ever made. It's because of your influence I know the kind of support and love to surround myself with.

To Matus: Thanks for playing with Dada while I was writing and editing this book. I hope I'm setting an example for you that working hard and being brave pays off. I will always support your dreams the way Grandpa and Dada have supported mine.

Lastly, to Grey: Words can't express how grateful I am for you and your unwavering support and confidence in me. Without your belief in my ability to be successful at whatever I pursue, I wouldn't be the person I am today. Thank you for loving me (and for putting up with not-infrequent outbursts and meltdowns as you challenge me to get out of my comfort zone).

ABOUT THE AUTHOR

Esther Avant, BS, CISSN, is a health industry veteran with over 18 years of experience in fitness, nutrition, and wellness related roles. She is a certified sports nutritionist, personal trainer, wellness coach, and owner of EA Coaching, which has provided full spectrum health and lifestyle coaching since 2015.

Her mission is to help women be healthy, happy, confident, and get the most out of their lives. She knows that if more women prioritized their health, they'd be able to unleash the confidence and focus they all need to leave their mark on the world.

Esther is also a boy mom and Navy wife who has lived and traveled all over the world while running her business.